JEAN FRENETTE'S

COMPLETE GUIDE TO

STRETCHING

JEAN FRENETTE'S
COMPLETE GUIDE TO
STRETCHING

BY JEAN FRENETTE

ⱳP

ISBN: 0-86568-145-7
Library of Congress Catalog Number: 89-051993

Designer: Danilo J. Silverio
Editor: Dave Cater

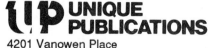

**UNIQUE
PUBLICATIONS**
4201 Vanowen Place
Burbank, CA 91505

TABLE
OF
CONTENTS

STRETCHING AND THE MARTIAL ARTS

No matter who you are or what your area of martial arts expertise, you'll never reach your maximum potential unless you incorporate a basic stretching program into your daily routine. I know plenty of forms and fighting competitors who lack the necessary flexibility to put themselves over the top. For a fighter, maybe he can't get his roundhouse kick out far enough to connect with his opponent. For a forms competitor, maybe he doesn't quite get the extension in his arms and legs to wow the judges. These may appear to be little things, but they can mean the difference between victory and defeat in a close contest.

Stretching and the martial arts go hand-in-hand, maybe more so than in any other sport. There is so much flexibility, so much suppleness required of the martial artist that to neglect this part of training would be to deny yourself the chance to realize your dreams.

First, stretching will help you achieve maximum comfort in your stance. A big plus for martial artists is to use your hips to the maximum and maintain a comfortable stationary position. Many times, if you're tight in the hip area you'll find it hard to generate power.

The visual results of a solid stretching program can be immediate and dramatic. You'll kick higher and with more power and you'll feel a better balance and control with your technique.This is especially true when training with a partner, because without the stretching program, every time you lift your leg you'll fall as he moves backward. But if you learn to stretch the right way, you'll soon see you can raise your leg higher and hold the leg longer.

Two weeks into your stretching you'll see a big improvement in your martial arts technique. You'll feel comfortable with yourself and your stance. This new level of achievement may not immediately be noticeable to your friends, but you'll know it. And best of all, you'll feel it. You have to search for results both inside and outside your body. Your body will give you signs, and if you follow a tested stretching program like mine, the results will always be positive. For those older people just starting the martial arts, a simple task such as walking will be an invigorating experience. You'll be stronger, have better balance and be more conscious of how your body and muscles work. For the first time in your life, you're learning to control your muscles. And what a great feeling it is!

Today I spend at least 20 minutes a day on my stretching routine. However, when I was working on the pre-stretching and beginners routine, I liked to work out at a maximum of 45 minutes. Everyone is different. If you're young, you might be able to handle a longer program. I'm a little older now so I don't push myself the way I used to.

I try to work on a day-on, day-off schedule. The day-on routine consists of heavy stretching. Here, anything goes. I try to isolate on the hips, with plenty of emphasis on the frog position. The day off is spent doing a light workout. Give your body a chance to recuperate and your muscles an opportunity to rejuvenate. For a change of pace I'll also do some running.

I never stretch the day after a competition, especially if I've had to perform both in the afternoon and evening sessions. The warm-up, cool-down, warm-up, cool-down schedule plays havoc with my muscles. I like to give them between 24-48 hours to bounce back. Also, if I'm competing I'll stretch both before *and* directly after the event to keep the muscles fresh and relaxed.

THE PHILOSOPHY OF STRETCHING

I started my martial arts training when I was nine and my first instructor, Maxime Mazaltarim, insisted that at least one-half of our workout should be spent on the specifics of stretching. Hungry as I was to get to the hard forms, I wondered what purpose a few twists and turns would have on my overall martial arts education.

Maxime could see the impatience in my eyes and assured me that everything we did, no matter how useless it might seem at the moment, had a fundamental purpose.

True to his word, about two-to-three classes later I began to notice a real difference in the way I felt. Suddenly the original tightness was gone, replaced by a new sense of movement. At the time I was playing a lot of hockey in my native Montreal, Quebec, and noticed I skated much more fluidly and actually felt stronger after stretching the day before. From that point I realized I could improve as much as I wanted if I only dedicated myself to stretching.

Of course, it was only natural for me to feel a bit of tightness in the beginning. My body and muscles were trying to adjust to a new way of life. Whether you're naturally flexible or very tight, you'll sense some stiffness. But that should only be momentary. After two or three classes, if you do good, solid stretching exercises, you'll feel a marked difference. At the outset, you may wonder if it's all worth it; your muscles are not used to being pushed to the limits. Given time, however, your body will adjust just fine. Remember not to force yourself. Patience is a virtue that pays high dividends in stretching. You're no good to yourself or your art if you get hurt. Learn to listen to your body; it will tell you when enough is enough. You cannot expect instant results. With any physical exercise where the frailties of the human body are involved, you must remember that we all are different. One person may progress quicker than the next. One person may recover faster. All in all, expect to see and feel the difference in approximately 14 days. It's good to set certain goals, but at the same time you have to be realistic. If you don't have patience, you'll soon become discouraged and quit. Now we don't want that, do we? I've been training for 18 years and among my peers I'm considered an expert. But I didn't achieve that status overnight. In fact, about three-to-four months into my training I experienced a series of peaks and valleys. I was careful not to press, not to push past what my body and mind were willing to do. Don't become overly discouraged if you stop improving at the earlier rate. Instead, take a couple of days off, relax and then return to your stretching regimen with renewed zeal and vigor.

3

HOW TO
STRETCH

We all know that one of the primary reasons for stretching is to prevent injury. As such, a few facts in the overall process should not be overlooked. One of the most common flexibility problems occurs in the lumbar region. Remember to maintain a straight back when you bend forward. This way you'll stretch both the back and leg muscles.

I also suggest a basic warmup session before you begin your stretching program. Tight, unprepared muscles are more rigid and difficult to stretch. A simple, five-to-ten minute warmup is sufficient to prevent a variety of injuries.

For some as yet unexplained reason, the greatest improvement can be realized when the stretching program is performed in the morning, usually a few minutes after rising. However, if this is not possible, an afternoon or evening program will suffice.

Although there are a variety of exercises, they can be grouped into three categories: dynamic stretching, static stretching, and negative stretching.

Dynamic Stretching

This is a fast repetition of an altering movement. In this instance, the muscle's spindle "senses" a rapid stretching of the muscles fibers' will, and in some circumstances, sends a signal to contract the stretch action. Since the action opposes the reaction, there is a definite potential for injury. To avoid this problem, I advise against using such exercises. Slow movement will trick the protection system, and therefore the contracting reaction of the stretched muscles.

Static Stretching

These exercises are performed slowly, bringing the body into a stretching position. The position is held for at least 20 seconds. Gymnasts are often seen "relaxing" while doing the "facial" split. You will feel the stretching stimulating, but after a while you will have to change position to regain that tension. Just remember not to change positions too quickly. The slow movements bring about the tension necessary for stretching without activating the muscle spindle, thus decreasing the chance of injury. It is for this reason I recommend this type of exercise over dynamic stretching.

Negative Stretching

This must *only* follow the static stretching exercise. Let's call the stretch muscles the protagonists and the opposing muscles the antagonists. First you place the muscles to be stretched (protagonists) in position (slowly) for about 20 seconds and then you contract the antagonists for five-to-ten seconds.

These exercises require the help of a partner who will block the body segment while you're contracting. After the contraction, you can relax and find yourself in the position to stretch more. Just as with static stretching, remember to move slowly and limit yourself to three-to-four contract relax sequences.

This type of exercise promotes rapid improvement in flexibility, but requires the help of a partner and takes longer to execute.

These are the basics on how to stretch. By following my recommendations, you'll notice a marked improvement without risking injury. Always remember to slowly execute the exercises and warm up before you start the program.

THE THREE POINTS OF STRETCHING

At all my seminars, I tell people that to write a stretching success story, you must always follow three key principles: maintain a solid lower back position; remember to concentrate; and breathe deep and easy to relax muscles. No matter how intent you are on learning the finer points of stretching, you are guaranteed never to achieve your ultimate goal unless you put the three aforementioned principles into practice. Let's discuss them individually:

Maintain a correct lower back position: This simply means keeping your lower back position straight at all times. In any exercise, whether you're on the floor, lying on your side or standing, your lower back will be directly involved in your movements. It is imperative to keep your lower back straight.

Why? Because every time you perform an exercise, your body will automatically shift forward. Most serious stretchers have a goal of touching their head to their knee. But this is wrong; you can achieve much more by maintaining a proper lower back position. But if you do it right, with the hips pushing forward and the lower back in perfect position, your abdomen will touch your thighs, your chest will brush your knee and your chin will touch your shin.

One common mistake made by many neophyte stretchers is to arch the back. But if you arch your back, your back will bend and that will detract from your stretch.

Let's suppose you're sitting on the ground with your legs extended. Your goal is to touch your toes or to touch your head to your shin. If you don't arch your back and rotate the hips first, your abs will touch your thighs, your head will touch your shin and your chest will rest against your knee. The muscle will stretch from the lower back to the tendon. However, if you keep your lower back straight, you'll feel the stretch from one end to the other. When the hips rotate first and the lower back position is maintained, you get the full benefit of your stretching exercise.

Concentrate on the area you're stretching: The successful bodybuilder is among the best athletes when it comes to concentrating on a particular aspect of the body. If he wants to work the biceps, he fashions his workout around the area in question. He has mentally fixed his mind on the area that needs work, thereby helping his muscle grow bigger and stronger. For example, if I'm stretching the groin muscle, I'm concentrating on the groin area because ultimately I want these muscles to be more flexible.

Learn to develop a mental attitude toward your stretching. By focusing your attention on a specific area, you will learn how to tell your body where you want it to go and feel the difference as it nears the final goal. Breathing helps you relax: When you breathe, oxygen flows through your body and into the muscles. This helps you relax and stretch to your maximum level. If you don't breathe slowly and deeply, you stand the chance of suffering cramps in the legs or abdomen area. Remember to inhale from the nose and exhale from the mouth. Concentrate and relax. Breathe in and out as you lean forward so you can relax the muscles.

THE
DANGERS
OF
STRETCHING

If you do follow my program to the letter, then you should stay clear of any major injuries. You'll reach your maximum potential without worrying about pulled muscles or other maladies. However, if you try to push yourself too hard, if you don't sufficiently warm up, or if you try to reach the next level too quickly, you may find yourself on the sideline wondering what went wrong. The result will be pulled and torn muscles or knee and ligament damage, all because you didn't take the time to learn the proper way to stretch.

In my many travels throughout the world, one of the biggest problems among martial artists is that they don't know how to stretch — correctly. To the majority, a proper stretching routine consists of five minutes of warmups followed by jumping around. Then they start throwing kicks. The problem is, while you may be ready to begin the hard training, your muscles are still ice cold. They're not ready to take the kind of constant pressure and pounding usually associated with martial arts forms.

Proper stretching will increase any martial arts movement, while decreasing the tendency for injury. Otherwise, you can expect to suffer knee, elbow, shoulder and hip problems. I've seen some guys hurt their ankle simply by throwing a side kick because they had not properly warmed up.

PRE-STRETCHING AND BEGINNERS LEVEL

Pre-stretching is for anyone who wants to prepare his body for the physical rigors that lay ahead. Whether you're a nationally ranked competitor or a neophyte with only a few weeks under your white belt, you need to gradually let your body and muscles stretch themselves, so when the real work begins they'll be prepared for the shock. It's kind of like starting your car and letting it run on a particularly cold morning. Driving it immediately could risk injury to the engine. It's the same way with your body. Give it a chance to warm up by breathing deeply to pump oxygen into the muscles.

If you've ever watched a sporting event, you'll always see athletes allow at least 15-to-20 minutes to stretch prior to the game. Sprinters such as Carl Lewis may take even longer, because a pulled muscle or tendon could hamper his performance for months. Pre-stretching, however, may be most important for martial artists. Many physicians claim the highly technical movements made by martial artists put undue stress on the body. With stress comes the very real risk of injury. That's why I emphasize pre-stretching. It's the easiest and most reliable way to help prevent injuries.

Although the pre-stretching routine only takes about 15 minutes, it can save you plenty of trouble down the road. One of the most important aspects of pre-stretching is *concentration*. You must always concentrate on the area you're trying to stretch. Remember to breathe slowly and deeply — inhale through the nose and exhale through the mouth. Feel the muscles relax as you stretch and breathe. Be careful not to bounce; this, too, will lead to injury. Simply go as far as you can and hold it. Take your time.

For those martial artists who compete on the tournament circuit, I suggest both the pre-stretching and beginners stages, as well as one or two of the intermediate exercises, just before hitting the floor. Do just enough to feel comfortable, but don't overdo it.

Neck Exercises

This "head rotation" exercise should be slowly performed, with the movement either right to left or left to right. Do it five times on each side. Start with the head rotation to the left (1). The head goes up (2) and then to the right (3). Move the head to the side (4) and finally down (5) to complete the circle.

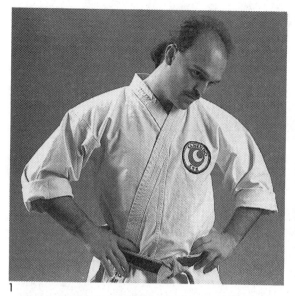

1

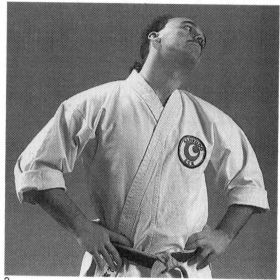

2

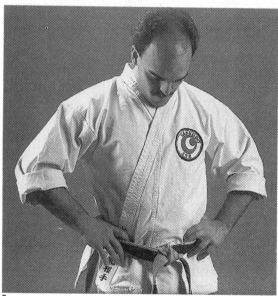

5

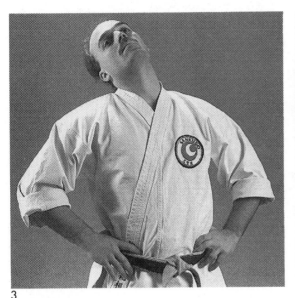

3

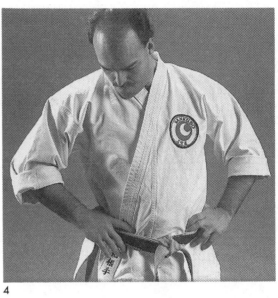

4

Hold the head straight (1). Move the head forward so the chin is on the chest (2). Slowly move the head backward (3). Do this ten times.

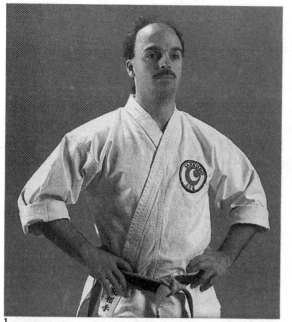
1

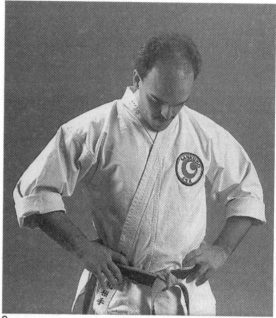
2

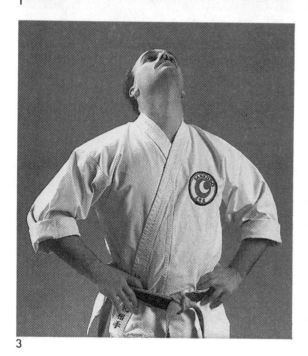
3

Hold the head straight (1). Tilt the head to the left in a relaxed manner (2). Now tilt it to the right (3). Do ten repetitions.

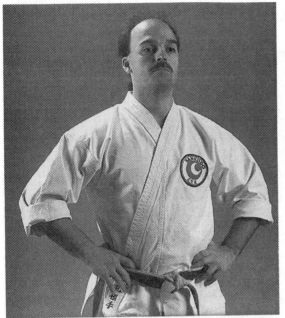

1

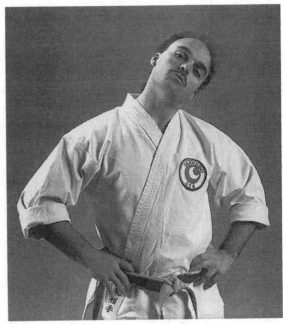

2

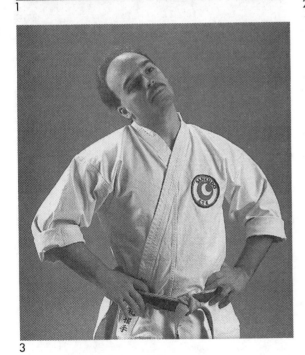

3

Shoulder Rotation

This shoulder rotation should be done both forward and backward. Be relaxed. Perform five repetitions. From a standing position (1), the shoulders should go up (2), back (3), all the way back (4), halfway down (5) and forward (6).

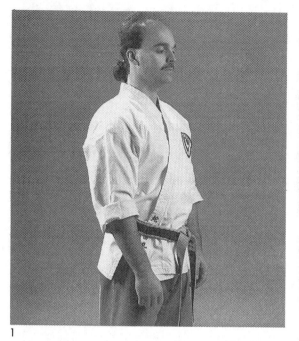

1

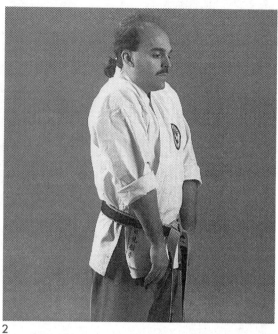

2

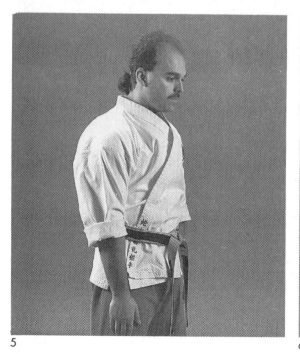

5

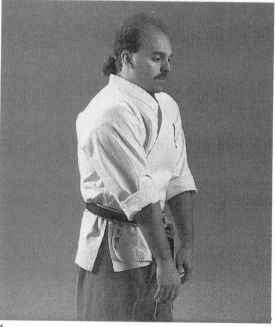

6

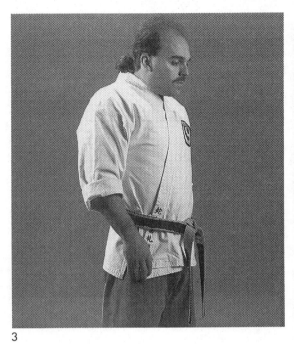

3

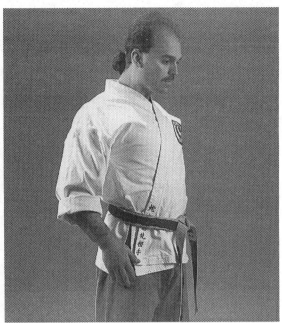

4

Arms Rotation

Keep your arms fully extended with your feet a shoulder-width apart. Perform 20 repetitions both forward and backward. Extend your arms to shoulder level (1). Start a downward rotation (2). Keep the rotations going in back (3). Rotate up straight (4), then forward (5) and finally back to the starting position (6).

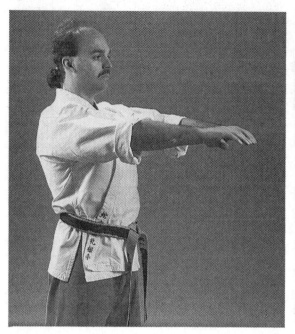

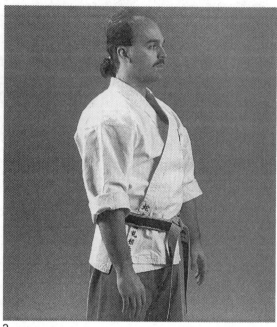

2

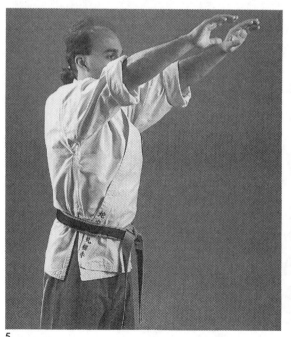

5

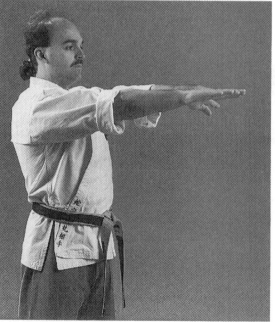

6

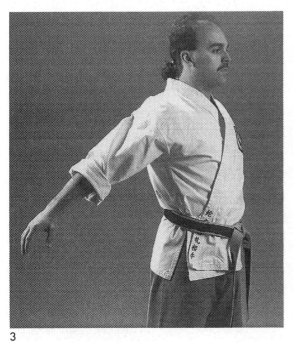

3

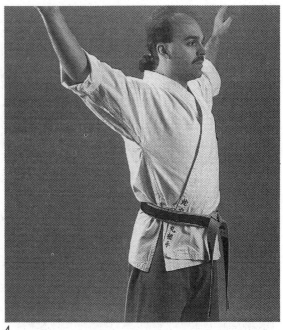

4

This shoulder exercise should be performed at normal speed. Do ten-to-15 repetitions. Extend the arms in front at shoulder level (1). Twist in your elbows, close your hands and slide on each side (2). Keep your elbows in and slide (3). Bring your elbows all the way back (4). Now bring back your arms in front with one relaxed movement (5).

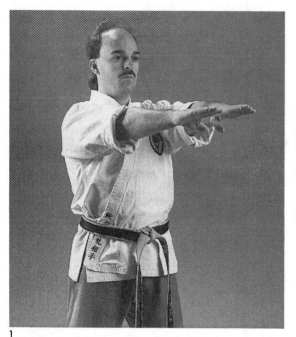

1

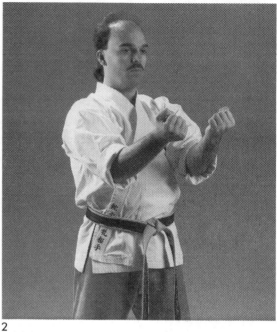

2

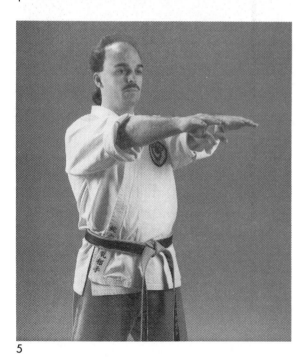

5

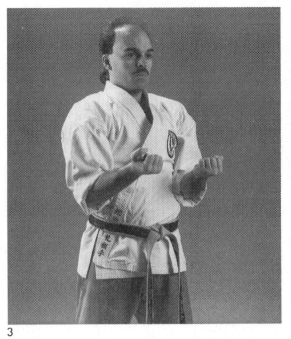

3

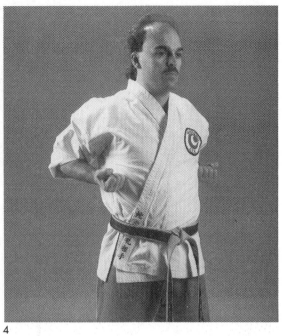

4

Perform this at regular speed, making sure to stretch as far as possible. Do ten-to-15 reps. Extend both arms in front (1). Open up your arms as though you are about to strike (2-3). Bring them back to center (4). Open up them again, fully extending the arms (5). Bring them back to the center (6).

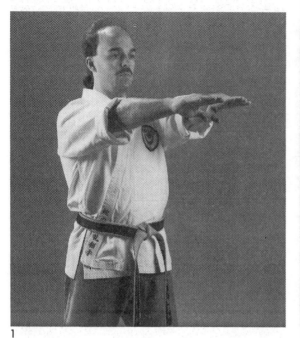

1

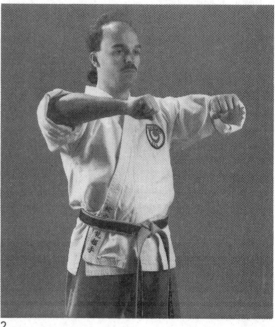

2

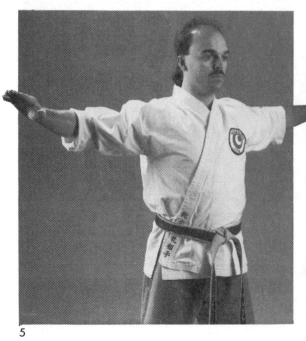

5

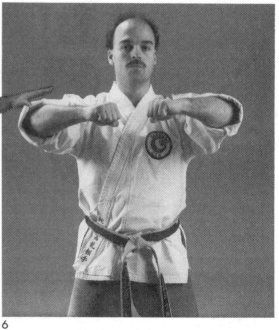

6

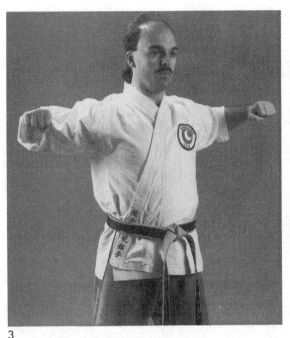
3

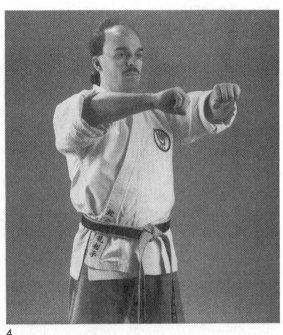
4

Lower Back and Spine

Do this exercise at regular speed. Perform 20 repetitions without stopping. Stand with elbows up and hands in the middle (1). Start twisting to the left (2). Keep turning to the left (3). Reach a maximum turn (4). Now turn to the right (5) until you've gone as far as you can go (6).

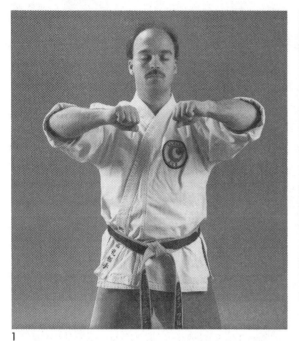

1

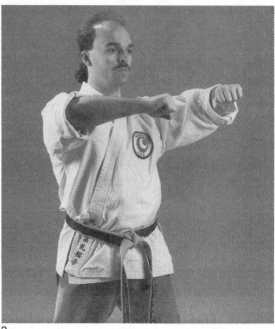

2

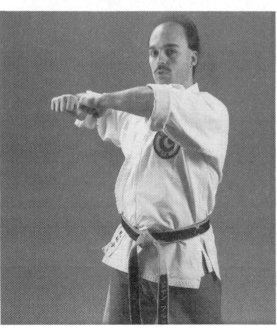

5

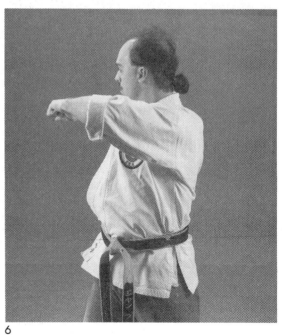

6

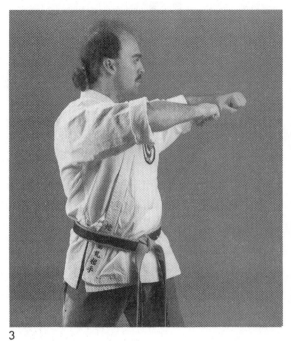

3

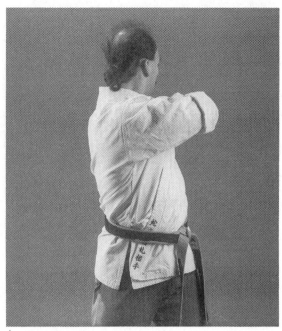

4

Hips Rotation

Start with your hands on your hips (1). Rotate to the left (2). Keep going forward (3). Then to center (4), and finally to the right (5). Move toward the front (6). Now return to the starting position (7). Do 20 full rotations.

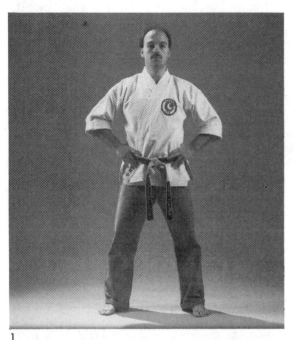

1

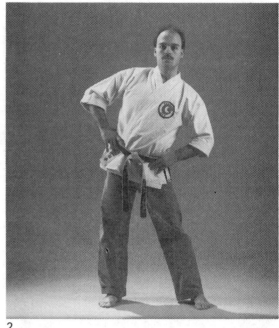

2

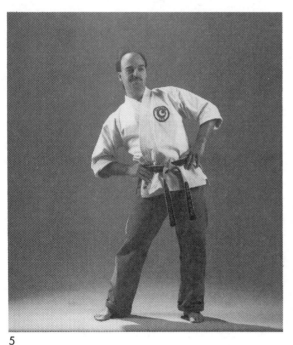

5

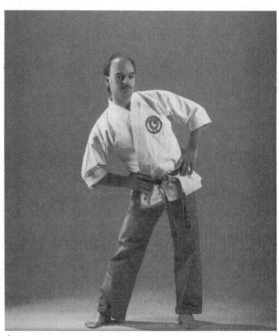

6

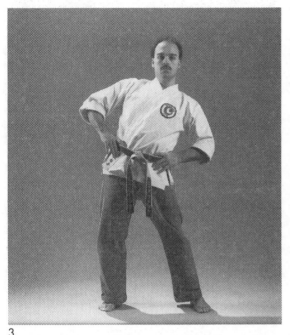

3

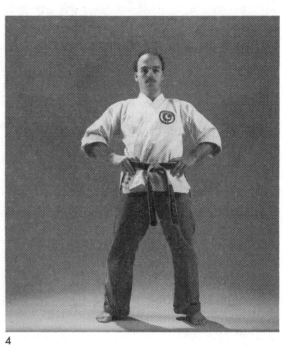

4

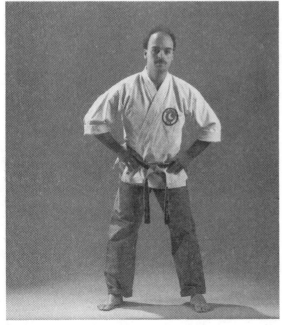

7

Spread feet three feet apart, with hands on hips and feet parallel (1). Start pushing hips forward (2). Push hips to maximum forward position (3). Then relax going backward (4). Be careful not to bend the knees.

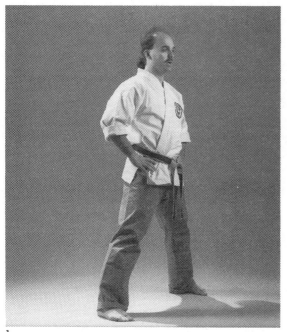

1

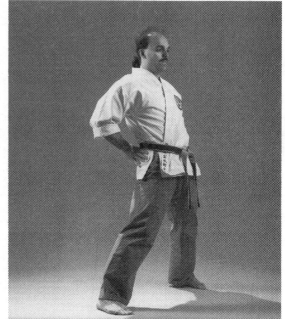

2

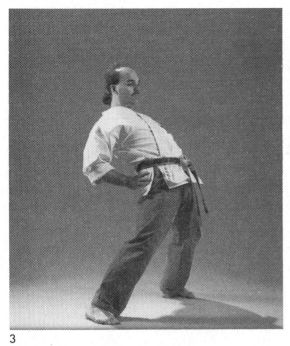

3

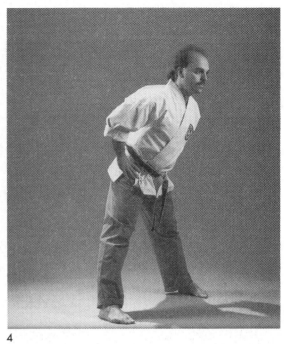

4

Hip Stretches

Spread legs three feet apart, with hands on hips and feet parallel (1). Start moving to the left, keeping your upper body straight and on line with the legs (2). Move all the way to the left (3). Return to the original position (4). Now do the same thing to the right (5). Move all the way to the right (6). Remember to exhale while stretching.

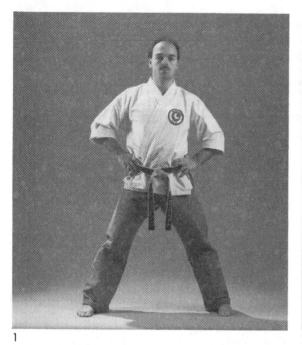

1

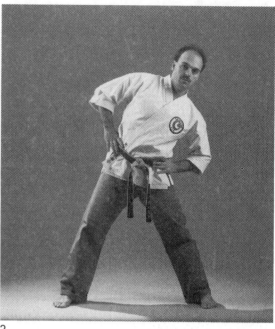

2

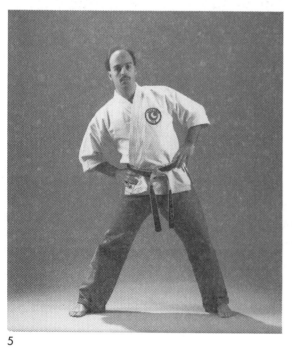

5

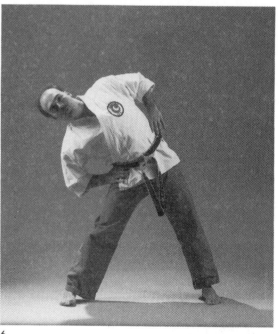

6

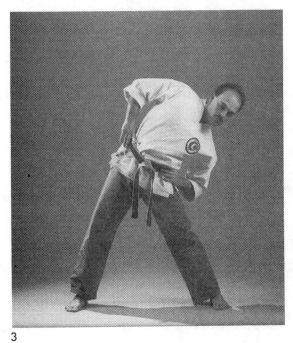

3

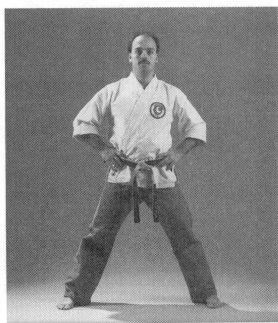

4

Spread legs three feet apart, with hands on hips and feet at a 45-degree angle (1). Start dropping with both knees square (2). Keep going down (3) until you can go no further (4). Do ten-to-15 repetitions and remember to keep the upper body straight.

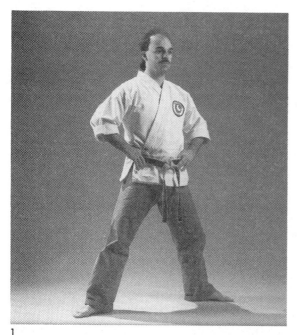

1

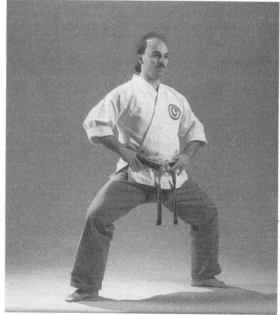

2

Assume a front stance (1). Start moving into a back stance (2-3). Now move into a stance where your front leg will be to the side and your toes will be pointing up (4). Keep the upper body straight.

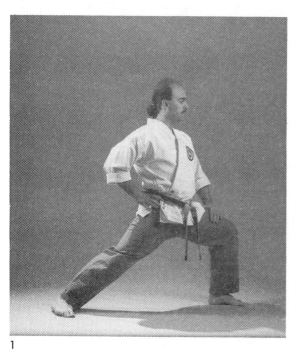

1

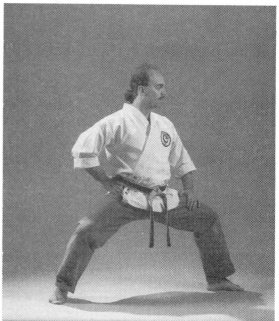

2

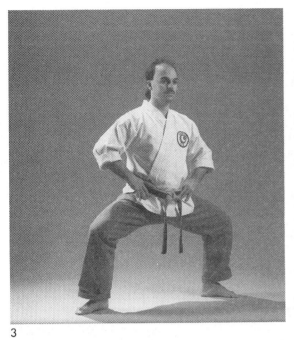

3

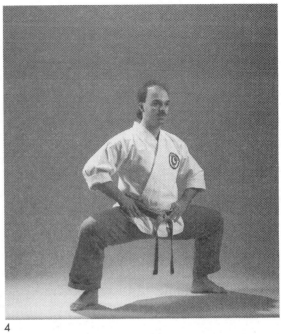

4

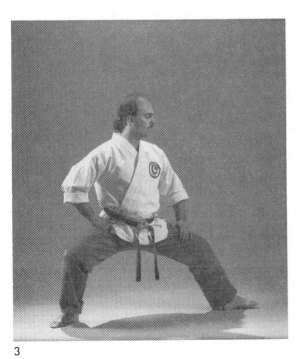

3

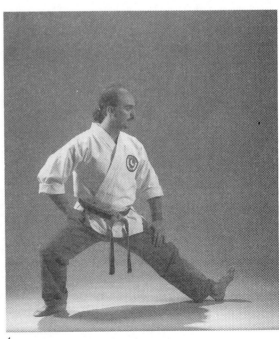

4

Spread legs three feet apart, with hands on hips (1). Start to bend the left leg, while keeping the right straight and in a side kick position (2). Go as far as you can (3). Return to the original position (4). Do ten-to-20 repetitions on both sides. The bending leg should have the knee facing in a 45-degree angle.

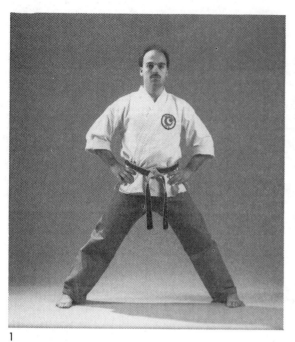

1

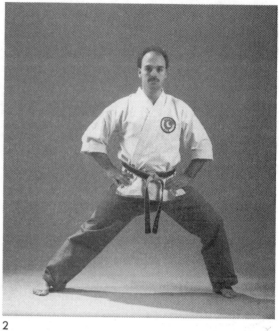

2

Leg Stretch

Spread legs three feet apart, with hands on hips (1). Twist to your right and slightly bend the knee (2). Bend all the way down (3).

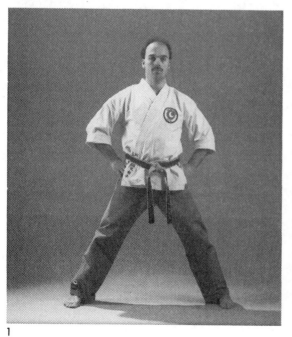

1

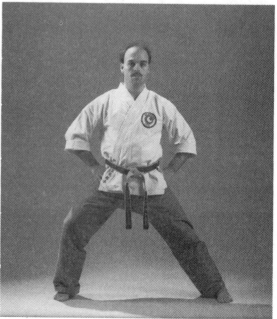

2

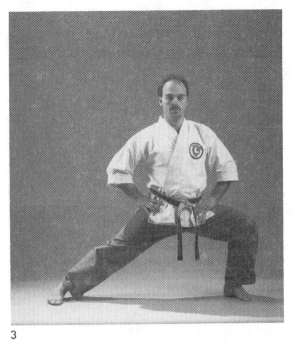

3

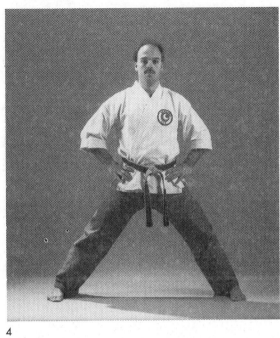

4

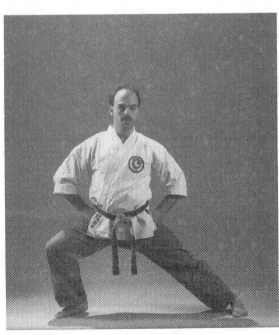

3

Spread legs three feet apart, cross your arms and keep your shoulders level (1). Start leaning forward, keeping lower back straight (2). Maintain a good position as you go down (3). Reach maximum and hold for ten seconds (4). Do three repetitions of ten, remembering to keep your lower back straight.

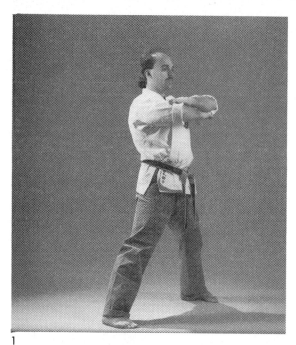

1

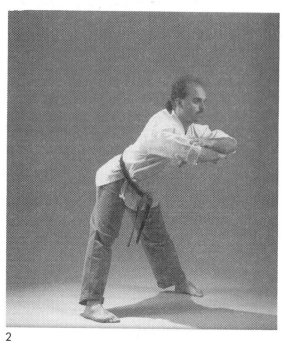

2

Start in the up position (1). Lift your left knee (2). Gradually bring your knee up to your chest (3). Hold this position for ten seconds (4). Do not bend the supporting leg.

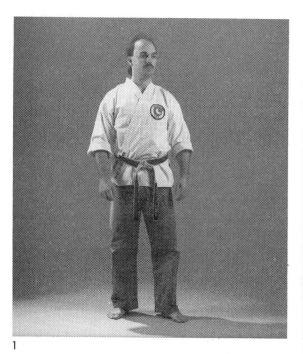

1

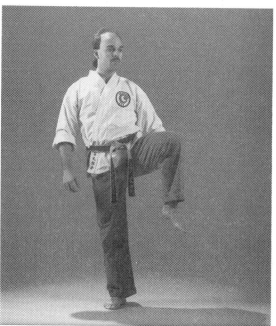

2

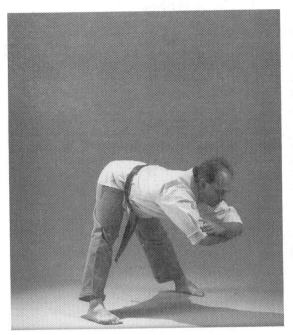

3

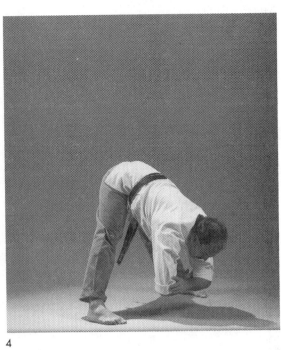

4

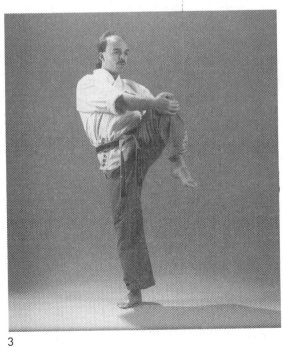

3

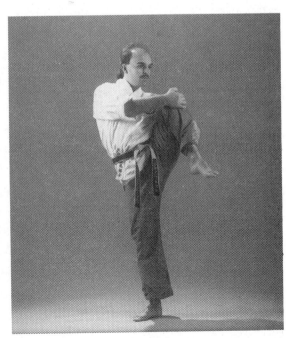

4

Sitting, extend left leg and bend the right (1). Keep your upper body straight. Start leaning toward your right knee, with your left leg in a front kick position (2). Go all the way to the ground (3). Hold this position for ten seconds (4).

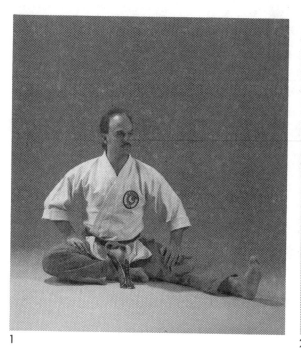

1

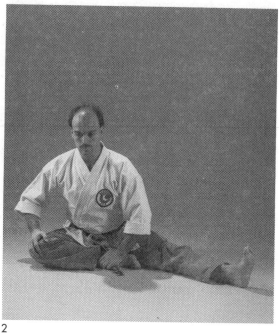

2

Sitting, extend left leg (1). Start leaning toward your toes (2). Keep going down (3). Go as far as you can and hold for ten seconds (4). Do this exercise three times, remembering to exhale as you lower your body.

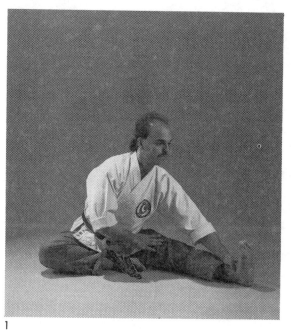

1

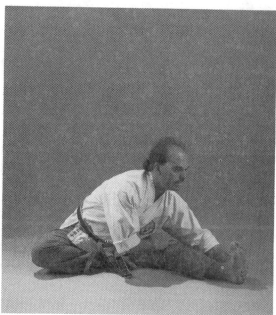

2

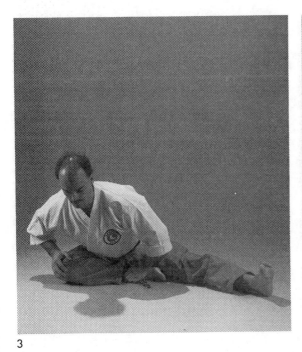

3

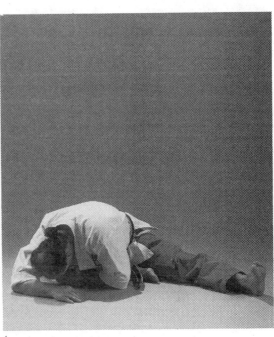

4

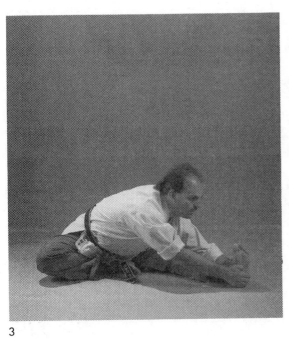

3

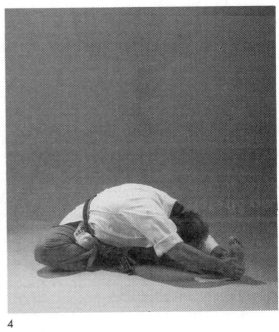

4

Sitting, extend both legs. Keep your back straight (1). Start leaning toward your toes, with the lower back making the first move (2). Keep moving toward your toes (3). Touch your toes (4).

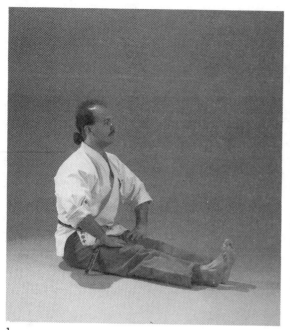

1

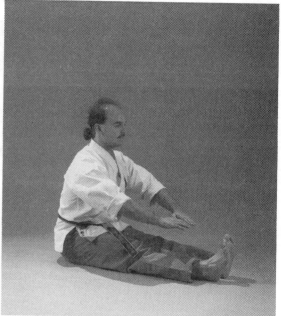

2

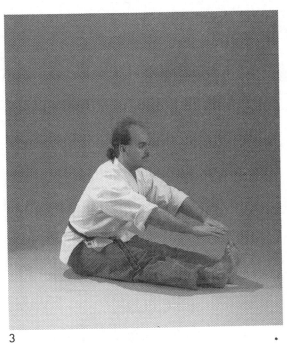

3

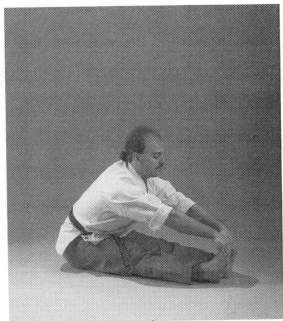

4

Sit down with your feet together as close as possible (1). Push down both knees (2-3) and hold for ten seconds (4). Now start leaning forward (5). The lower back will make the first move. When you've gone as far as you can, hold for ten seconds (6). Do three sets.

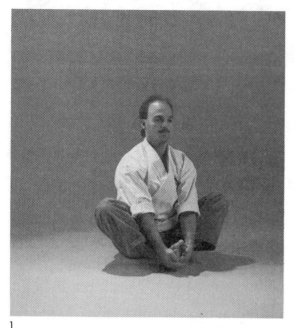

1

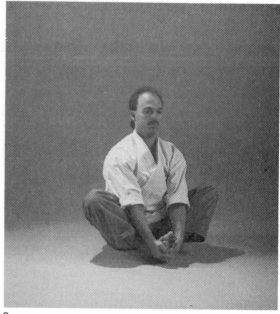

2

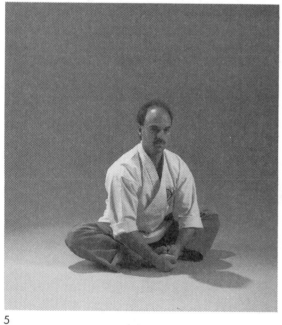

5

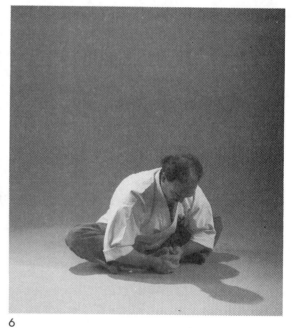

6

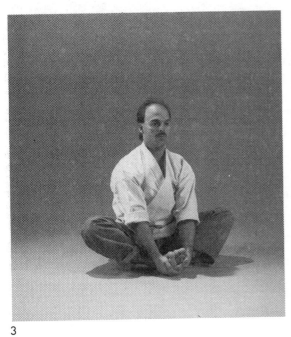

3

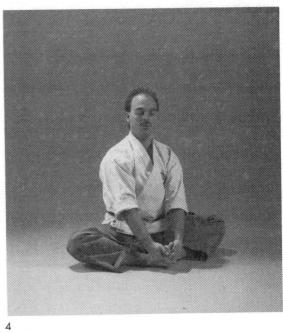

4

Sit with your legs as open as possible without hurting (1). Move to the left, keeping your upper body straight (2). Go only halfway (3). Return to first position (4). Slowly go to the right (5). Go only halfway (6). Return to the first position (7). Do 20 repetitions and hold each for two seconds.

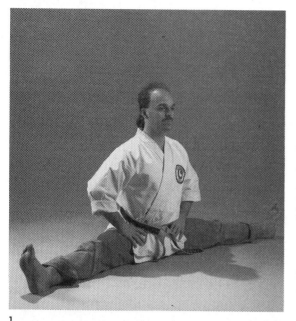
1

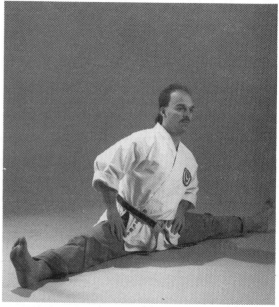
2

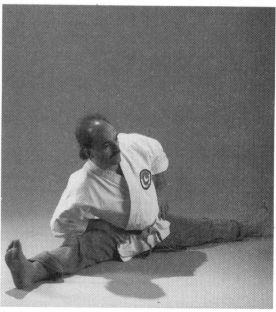

5

6

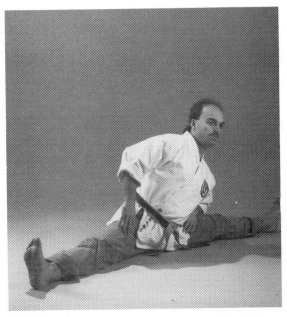

3

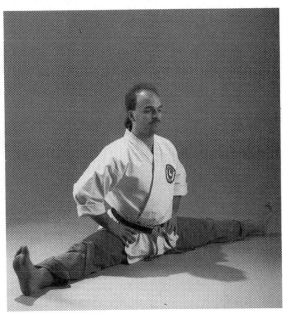

4

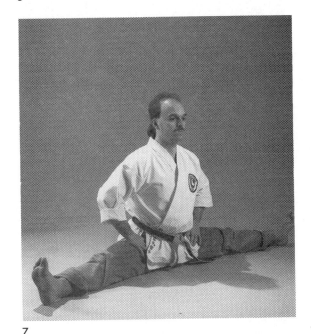

7

Leg Stretch

Sit with your legs as open as possible and your toes pointing up (1). Touch your toes (2). Move to the right and touch your toes (3).

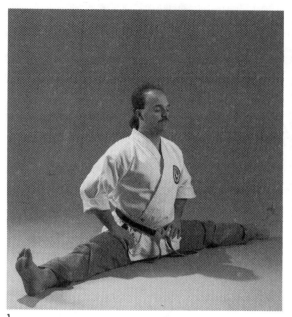
1

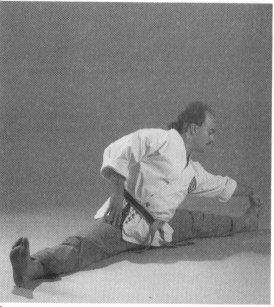
2

Sit with your legs as open as possible (1). Start forward with your hands on the floor (2). Keep going forward (3). Rotate the hips forward (4). Reach as far as you can and hold for ten seconds. Do a minimum of three repetitions. Concentrate on the hips and groin muscle.

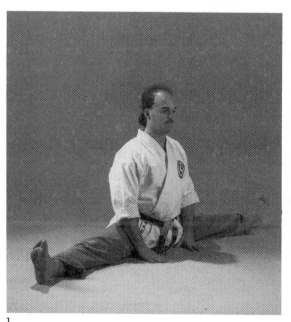
1

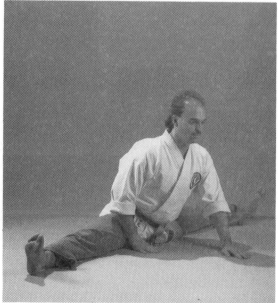
2

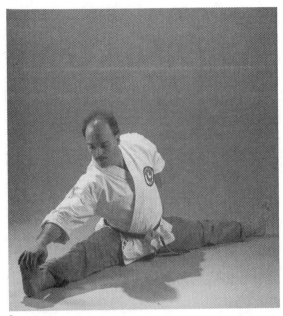

3

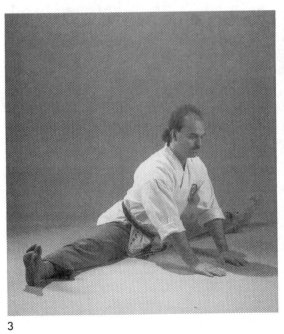

3

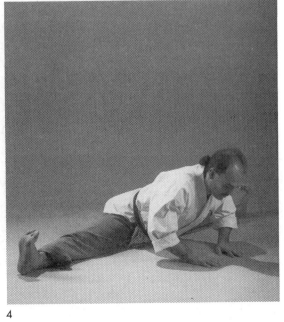

4

Knee Stretch

Stand straight (1). Bend both knees halfway (2), keeping your hands on your knees. Circle your body right to left (3). Do this slowly, with your knees at the same level (4). Execute circle motion (5). Finish the circle and reverse the motion (6). Do ten circles on each side.

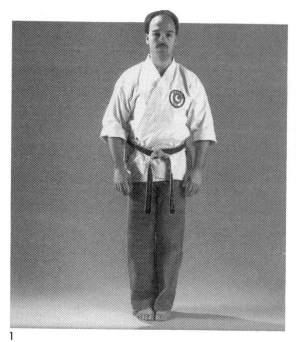

1

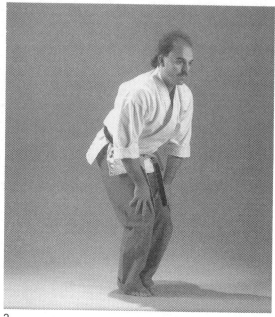

2

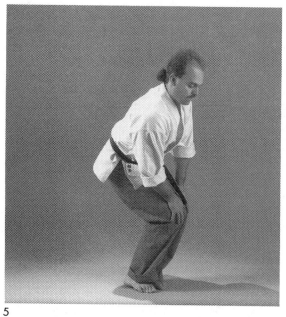

5

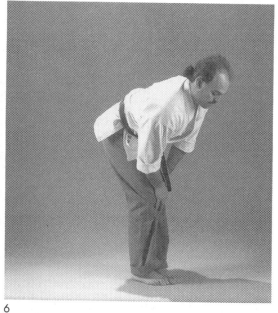

6

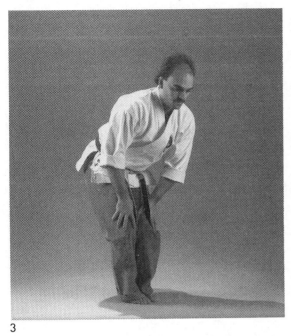

3

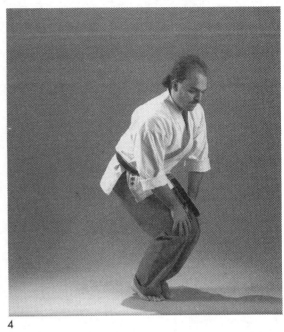

4

Leg Stretch

Sitting, extend both legs (1). Lean, grab your feet and pull so heels come off the floor (2). Pull more to stretch the calf tendon (3). Lean forward as far as possible and hold for five seconds (4). Perform three repetitions.

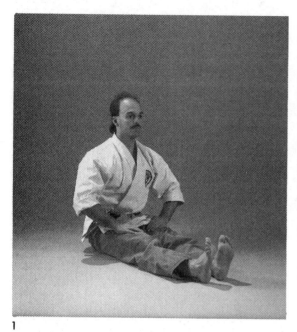

1

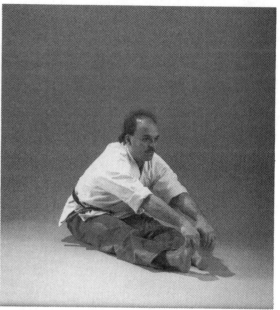

2

Sitting, bring your knees to your chest and grab your feet (1). Extend your left leg as high as it can go and hold it for five seconds (2). Do the same with the right leg (3). Perform three repetitions with each leg.

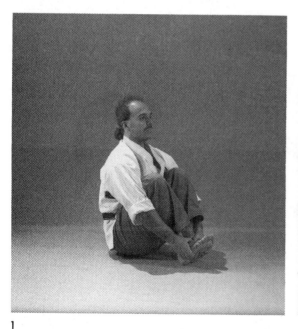

1

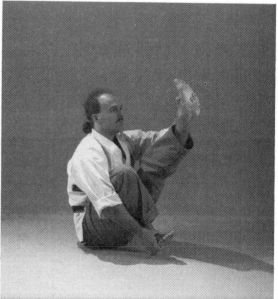

2

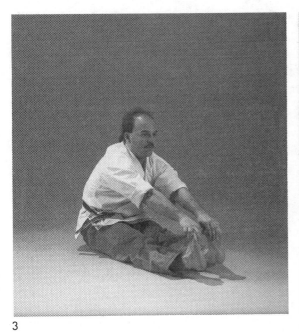

3

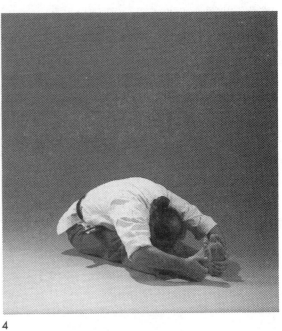

4

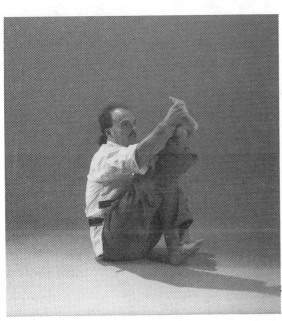

3

Extend left leg as far as you can. The right leg is bent inside (1). Lean forward so the right foot touches your belt (2). Move to the left and touch your head to your shin (3). Do three repetitions of each, holding it for ten seconds.

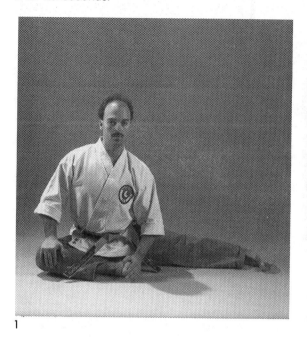

1

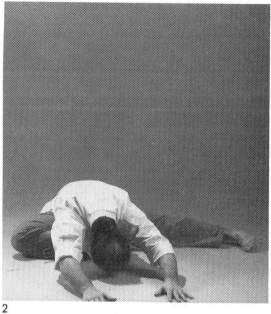

2

Sit with legs open as far as possible (1). Lean forward as far as you can (2). The arms are straight in front. Spread arms and hold for ten seconds (3). Move to the left and touch your head to your shin (4). Hold for ten seconds. Do the same thing on the right.

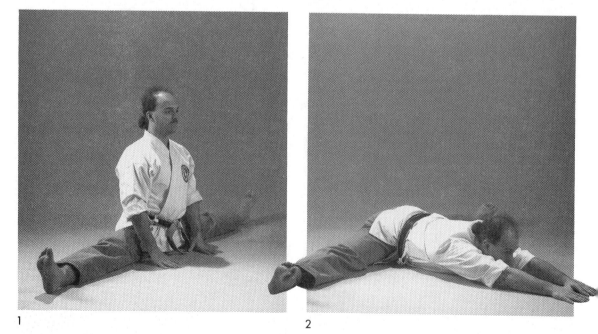

1

2

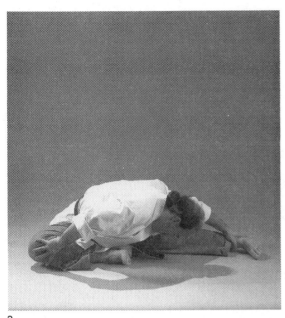

3

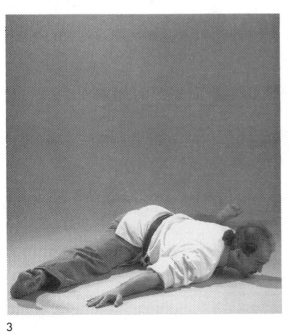

3

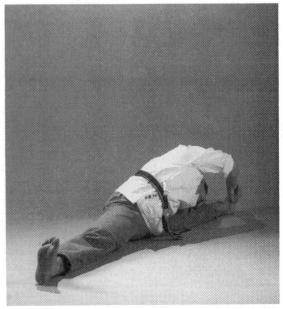

4

Extend left leg in a front kick position (1). Lean forward and touch your head to your shin (2). Hold for ten seconds. Turn toward your opposite knee and hold for ten seconds (3). Remember to keep a straight line with the left leg, hips and right knee. The right heel should be touching your buttocks. Do three repetitions for each leg and each side.

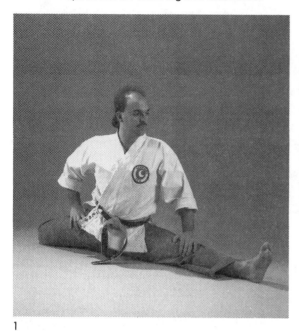

1

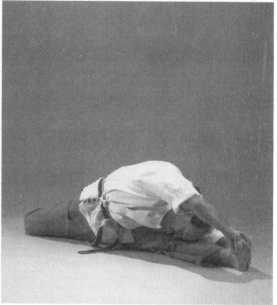

2

Mid-Air Stretch

Stand with your legs three-to-four feet apart (1). Drop your head to your left shin and hold for ten seconds (2). Now perform the same move on the right side (3). Finish with a forward bend, grabbing both ankles. (4).

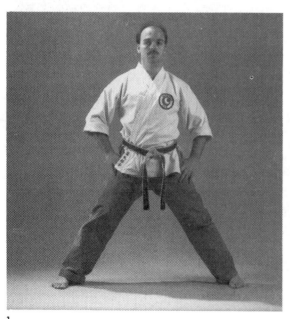

1

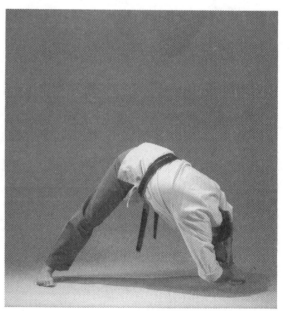

2

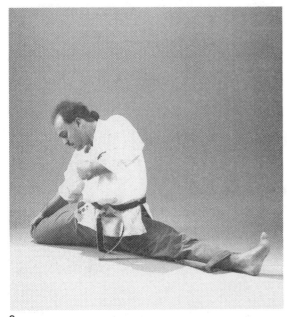

3

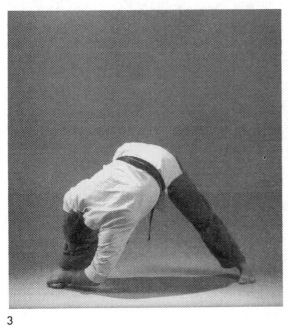

3

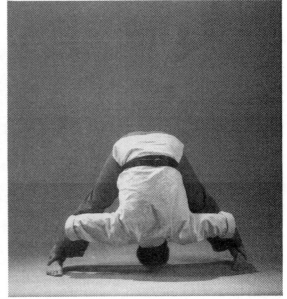

4

Partner Stretching

Sit with both legs extended and a partner behind (1). As your partner pushes your back, you reach out to grab your toes (2). Go as far as you can and hold for ten seconds (3). Do two repetitions.

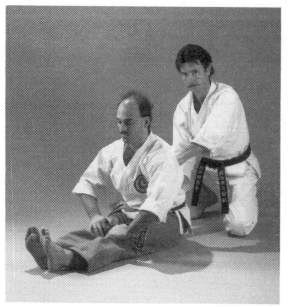

1

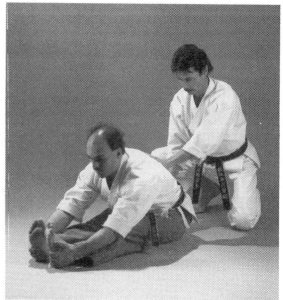

2

Sit in a butterfly stretch with your partner behind (1). Your partner puts pressure on your lower back with his shoulder and knee (2). Go as far as you can and hold for ten seconds (3). Do two repetitions.

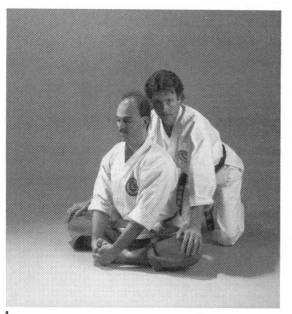

1

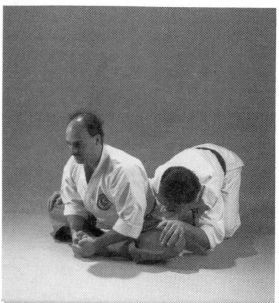

2

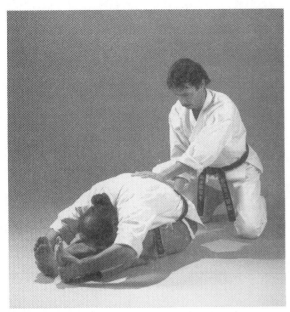

3

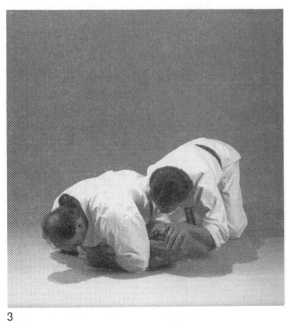

3

Sit with legs apart as far as they will go. Your partner is behind you (1). Your partner pushes your lower back while holding your knees (2). Go as far as you can and hold for ten seconds (3). Do two repetitions.

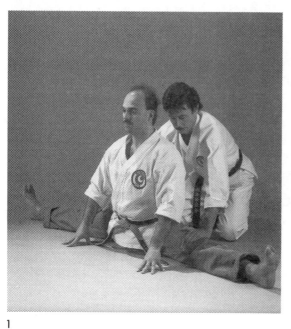 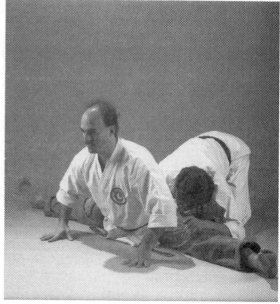

1

2

Do a butterfly stretch on your back (1). Your partner is holding your knees. As your partner pushes down, keep your head up (2). Hold final position for ten seconds (3). Do two repetitions, keeping the knees as close as possible to the groin.

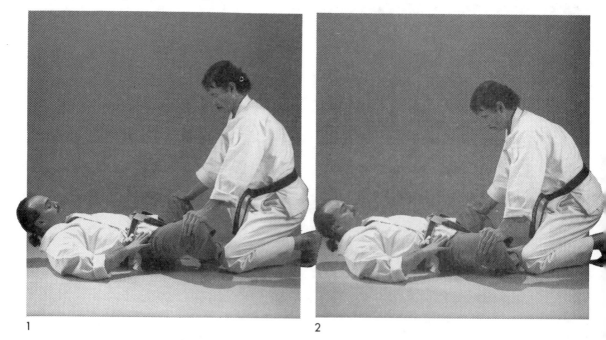

1

2

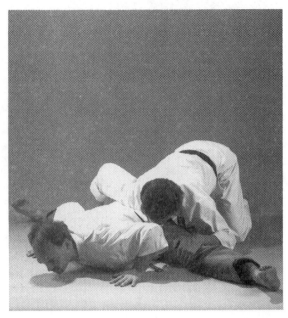

3

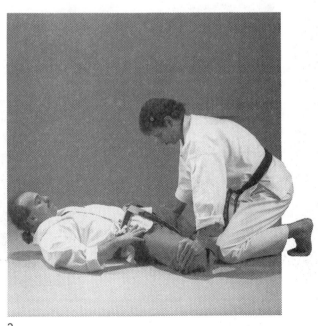

3

Assume a deep front stance for ten seconds (1). Start moving backward (2). Reach as far back as you can go (3). Keep your upper body straight. Be careful not to lean.

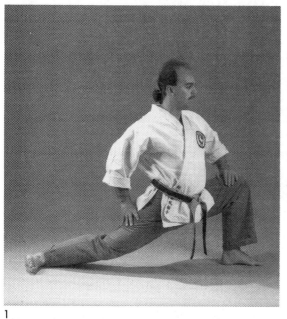

1

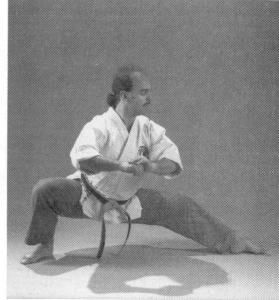

2

Stand with feet three feet apart and grab your ankles (1). Bend the right leg while the left is kept straight (2). Go as far as you can and hold for ten seconds (3). Do this 20 times on each side.

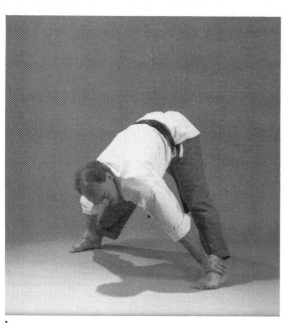

1

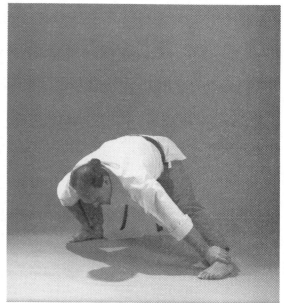

2

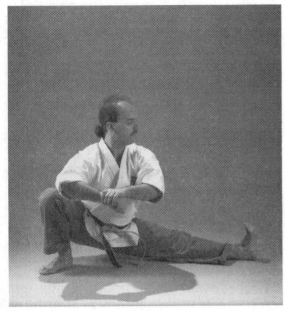

3

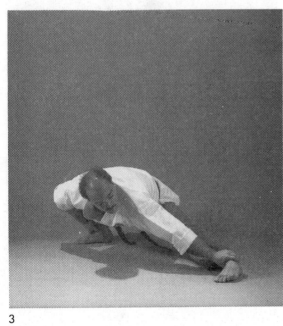

3

Place your front knee on your partner's shoulder (1). Your partner moves back (2). Hold this position for ten seconds. Do three repetitions.

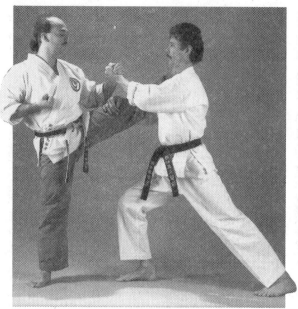

1

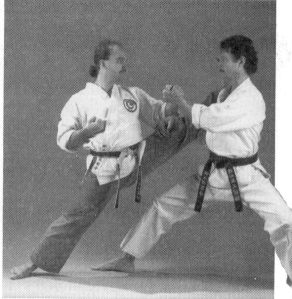

2

Assume a side kick position and place the leg on your partner's shoulder (1). Your partner moves back (2). Hold this position for ten seconds and repeat three times.

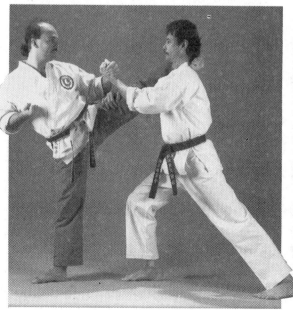

1

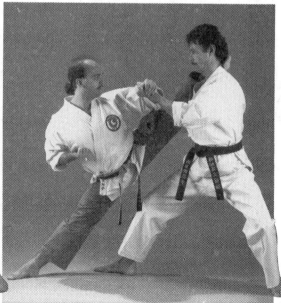

2

Assume a back kick position and place your leg on your partner's shoulder (1). Your partner moves back (2). Hold this position for ten seconds. Do three times.

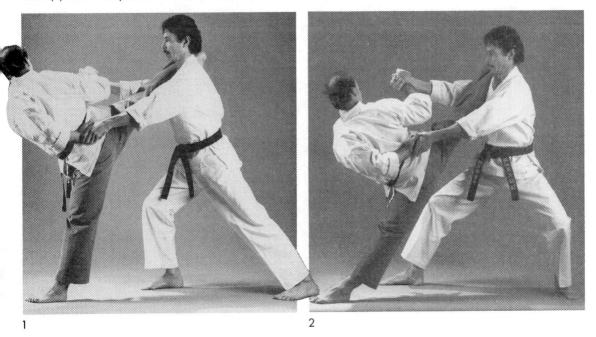

1

2

If you cannot put your leg on your partner's shoulder, have him grab your leg at waist level (1-2).

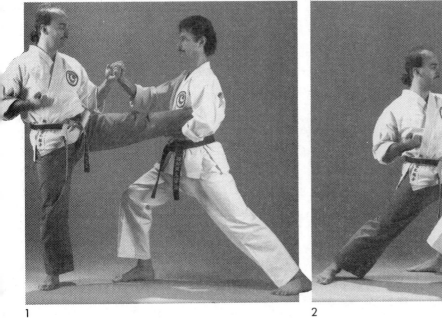
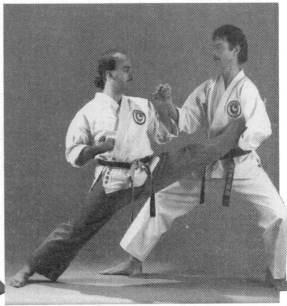

1

2

Sit on the floor with your legs open (1). Your partner is holding your belt. Your partner starts pushing with his legs and pulling your belt (2). Go as far as you can and hold for ten seconds (3). Repeat twice.

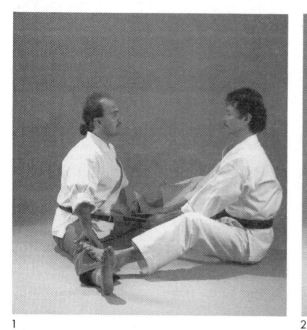 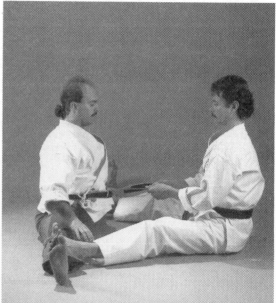

1   2

Assume a front kick position with the partner behind you holding your lower back (1). Have the partner in front lift your leg (2). Have him move the leg as far as he can and hold for ten seconds (3). Do two repetitions.

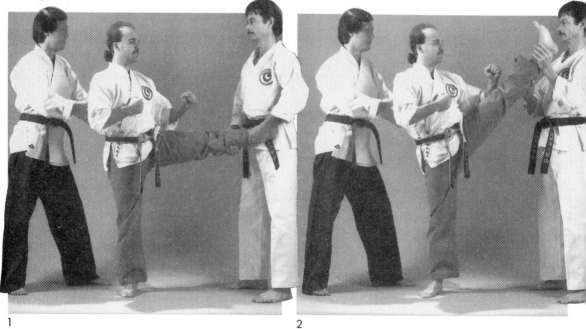

1   2

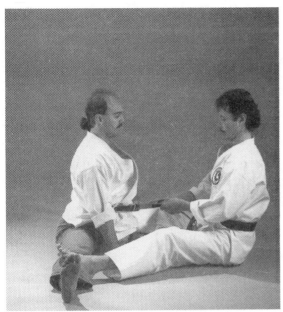

3

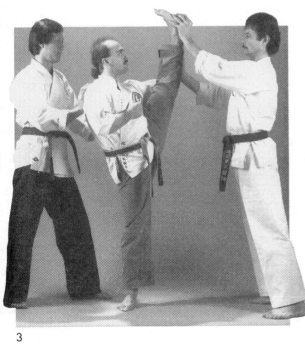

3

Two-Partner Stretching

Assume a side kick position (1). Have him push up on your right leg (2). Go as far as you can (3). The partner behind you should hold you in a solid position. Hold for ten seconds.

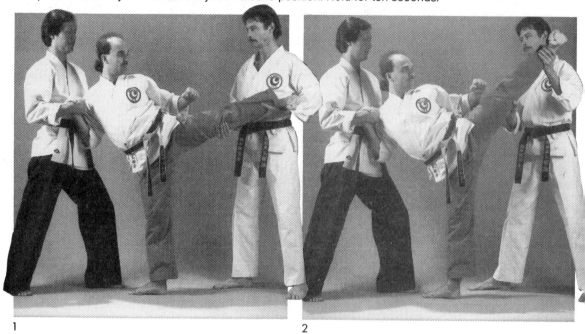

1

2

This exercise is the same as the side kick two-partner stretch except you are using the back kick (1-4).

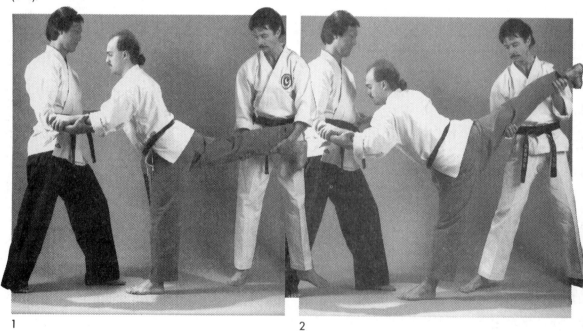

1

2

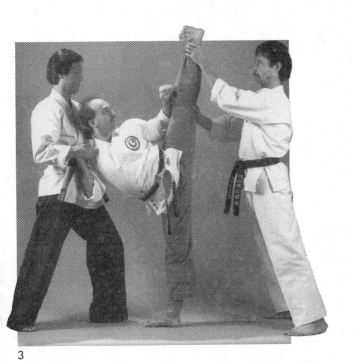

3

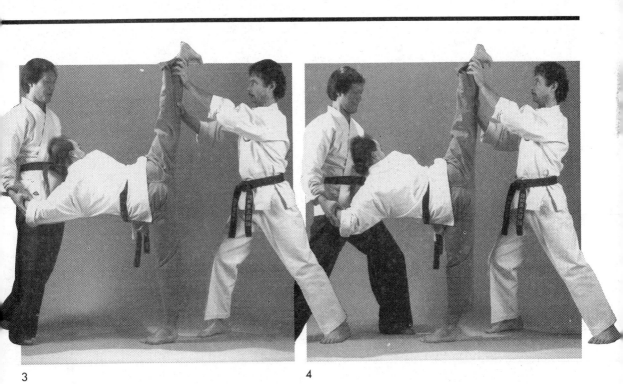

3   4

INTERMEDIATE STRETCHING

While the pre-stretching routine is for everybody, no matter how flexible you are, the intermediate level is reserved only for those practitioners who have had some previous stretching experience.

To tell if you are ready to move on to the next stage, try this simple experiment: Perform every exercise in the pre-stretching and beginners routine. Try to take it to the maximum. If it pulls but doesn't burn when you take it either very high or very low, you are ready for intermediate stretching. The rule of thumb is that if you feel like you can push more, it's time to go on. At this secondary stage, you can do the beginners exercises with ease. You can touch your shoulders to the ground and every knee stretch won't appear difficult enough.

While on your back, raise both legs and grab the inside of the knees (1). Start to spread your legs (2). Stretch as far as you can (3). Hold for ten seconds. Do three repetitions.

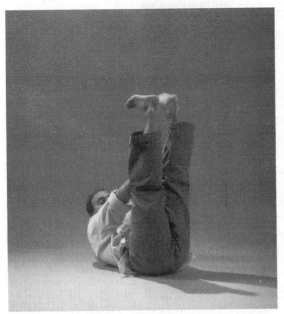

1

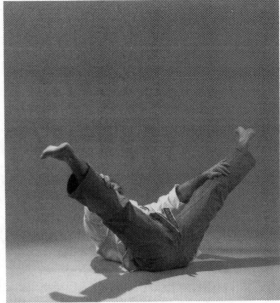

2

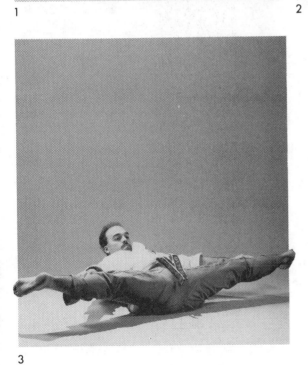

3

Assume a right leg front stance (1). Twist your hips to the right (2). Now lift your left leg to the right side (3). Bring the leg all the way up (4). Begin moving the left to the left (5). Drop the left leg (6). Return to the first position (7). Do ten reps on each side.

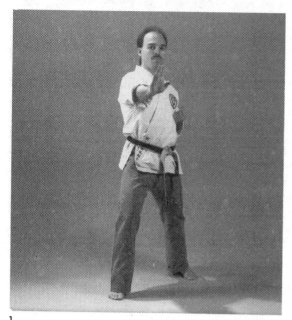

1

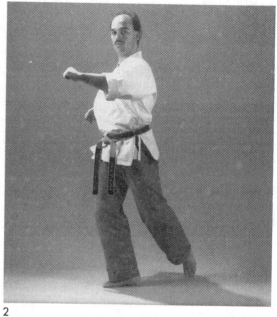

2

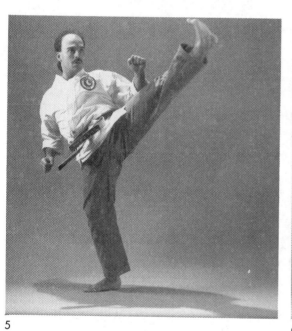

5

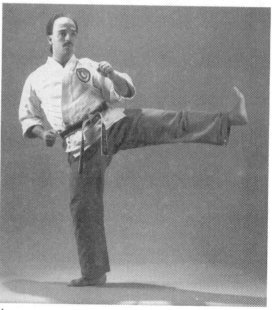

6

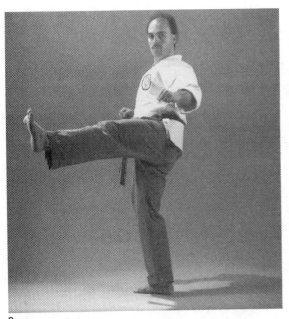

3

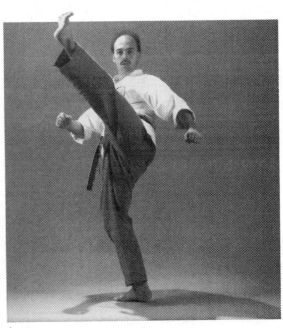

4

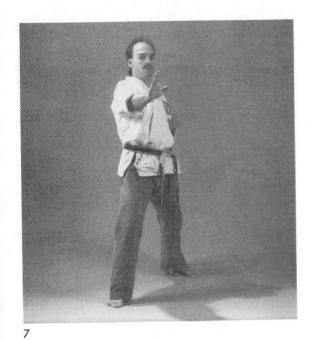

7

Face the floor, with both knees behind and back straight (1). Go straight down, with your back legs at a 90-degree angle (2). Hold for ten seconds. Move backward and hold for ten seconds (3). Move forward and hold for ten seconds (4). Extend your right leg in a side kick position (5). Go down and hold for ten seconds (6). Repeat twice.

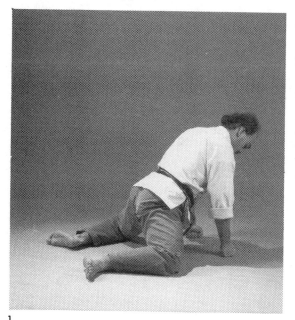

1

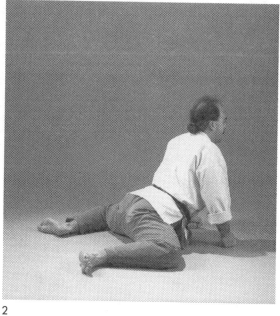

2

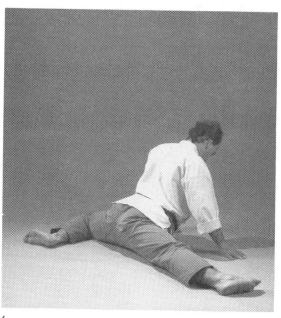

5

6

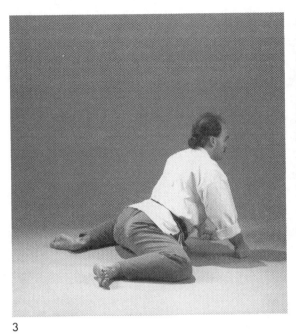

3

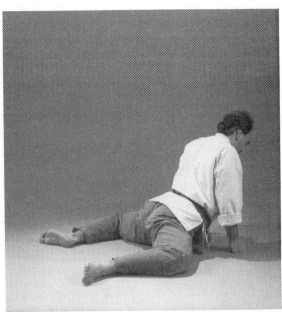

4

Partner Exercises

You are on your back with both knees up. Your partner has locked his knees with yours (1). Your partner pushes down on your knees (2). Go as far as you can and hold for ten seconds (3). Extend your left leg in a side kick position (4). Your partner pushes down on the leg (5). When you've reached as far as you can go, hold for ten seconds. Then relax (6). Now extend both legs (7). Your partner pushes down both legs (8). Hold for ten seconds when you can go no further. Do twice and exercise both legs.

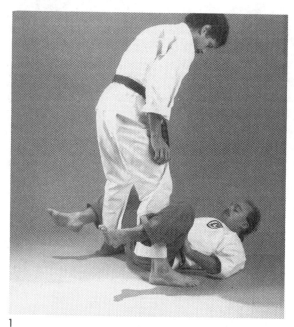

1

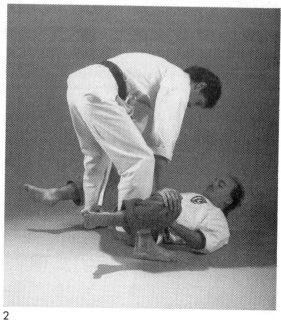

2

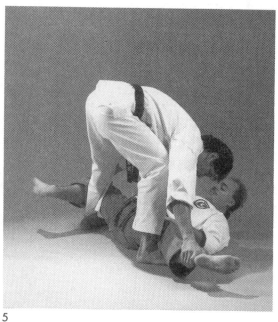

5

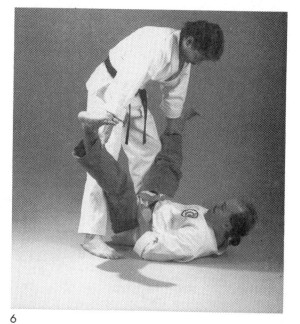

6

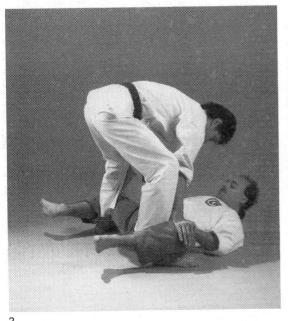

3

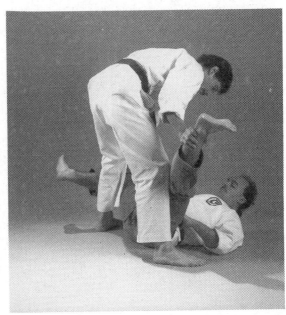

4

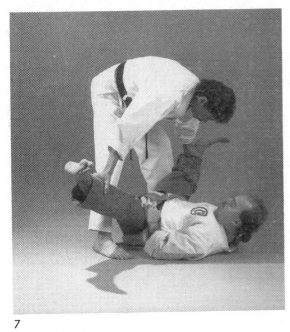

7

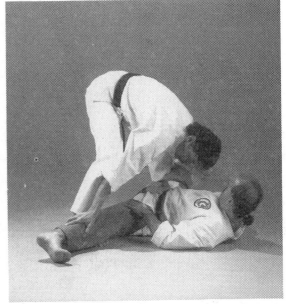

8

Lie on your back and bring your feet together inside to your groin (1). Your partner will push your knees down all the way (2). Remember to keep your head up.

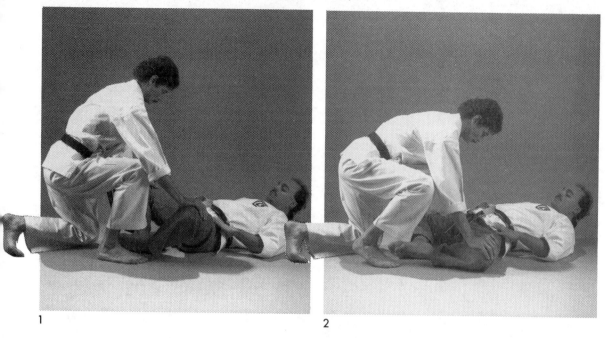

1

2

Side Stretch

Lie on your right side and extend your left leg (1). Your partner slowly lifts your knee (2). Go to the maximum and hold for five seconds (3). Do two repetitions of five seconds on each side.

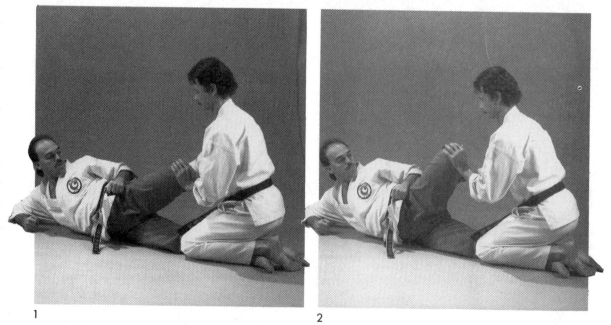

1

2

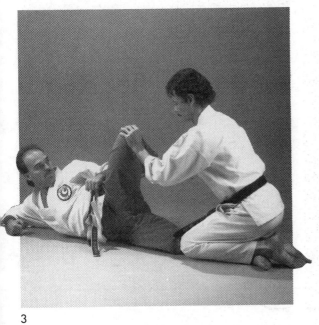

3

Assume the frog position (1). Your partner pushes straight down on your hips (2). Next extend your left leg while your partner pushes down on your hips (3). Hold for five seconds.

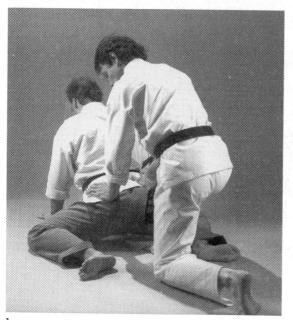

1

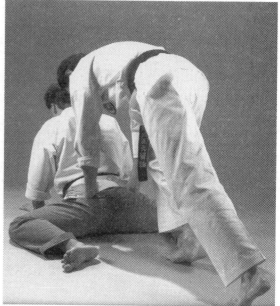

2

The right leg is bent and the left leg extended (1). Twist into a right leg deep front stance (2). Go back and extend the right leg while bending the left (3). Twist into a left leg deep front stance (4). Continue the action for five complete sets.

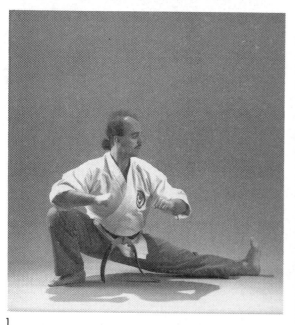

1

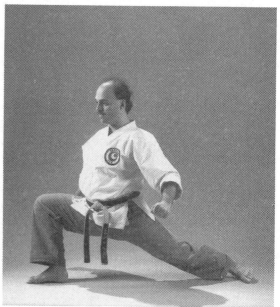

2

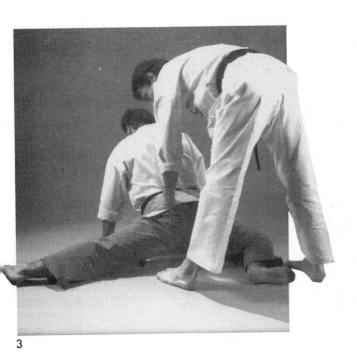

3

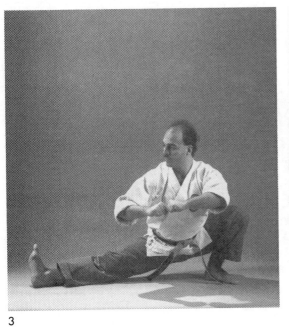

3

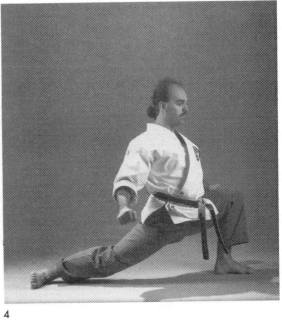

4

Assume a deep front stance position (1). Move back (2-3).

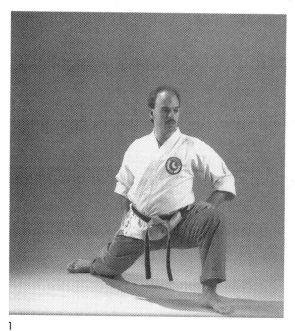 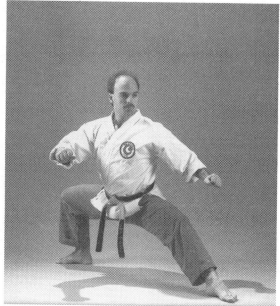

1   2

Hips Rotation

This is a right leg bend with the left leg in an extended front kick position (1). Dip and stretch as much as you can (2). Hold for ten seconds.

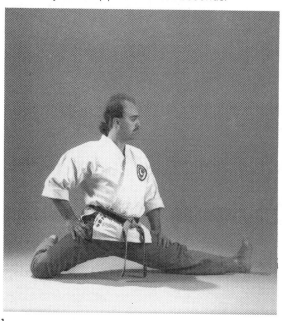 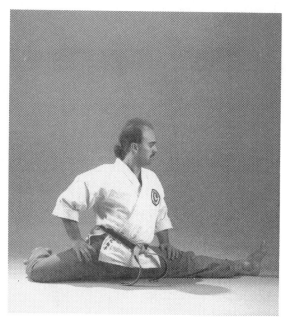

1   2

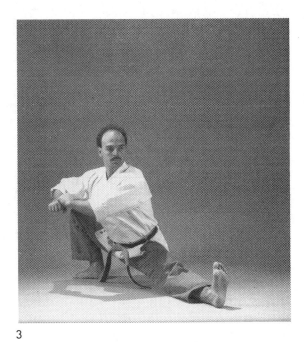

3

Get into a full splits position (1). Start pivoting the hips forward (2). Pivot as far as you can and hold for three-to-five seconds (3).

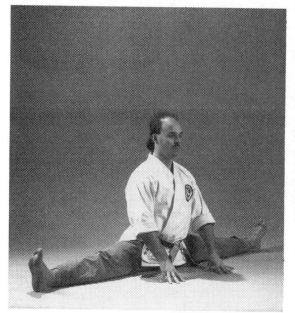

1

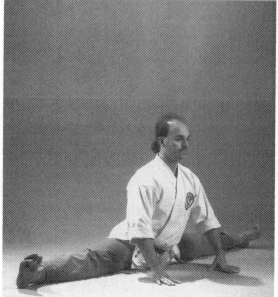

2

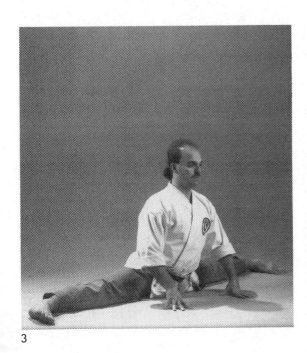

3

Isometric Exercises

Assume a butterfly position with your partner pushing down (1). Try to bring your knees together (2). As your partner offers resistance, push hard (3). Now try to pull your knees apart (4). Make sure your partner is giving plenty of resistance (5). Go as far as you can (6). Hold for three seconds (7). Repeat twice.

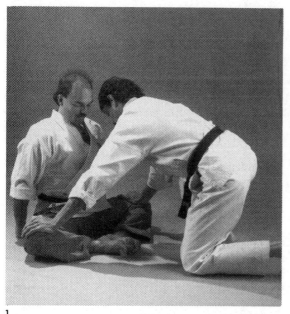

1

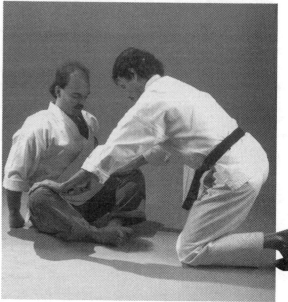

2

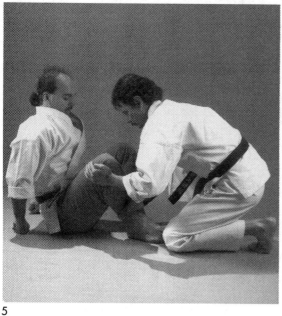

5

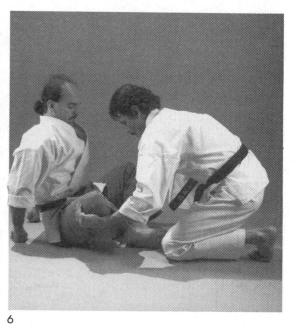

6

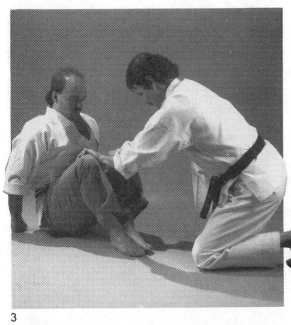

3

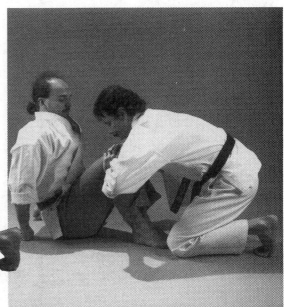

4

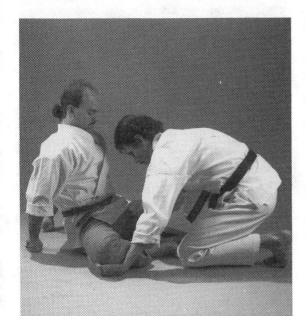

7

You are on your back, feet together (1). As your partner offers resistance, try to bring your knees together (2). Keep pulling up without taking a break (3). Your partner places his hands on the outside of your knees (4). Try to open your legs (5). Try to touch your knees to the floor (6). When you've gone as far as you can, hold for three seconds (7). Remember to keep your head up and concentrate on the groin muscles.

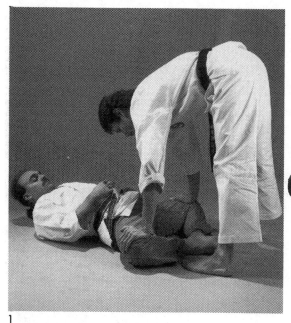

1

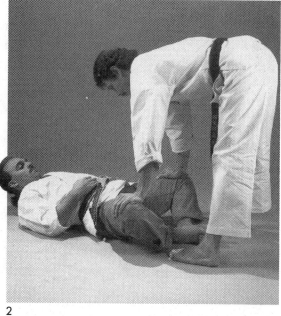

2

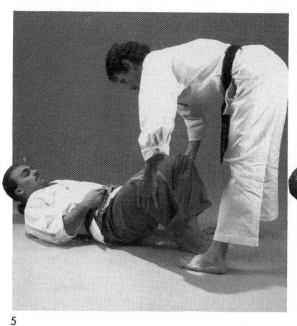

5

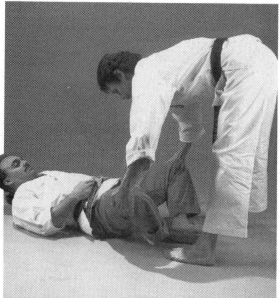

6

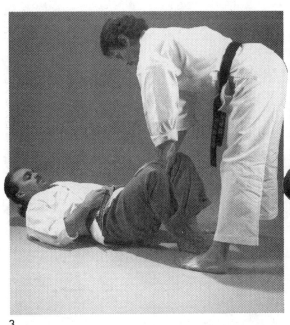

3

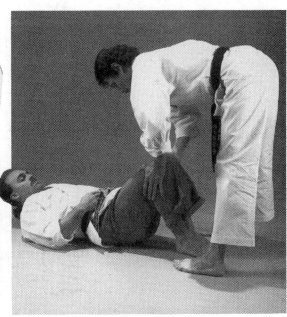

4

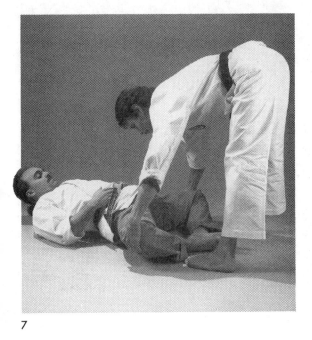

7

You are on your back, knees up straight and in line with the hips (1). Try to bring the knees up as your partner resists (2). Go as far as you can and hold for three seconds (3). With your knees together, try to open them as your partner resists (4). Keep opening, making sure your head is up (5). Go as far as you can (6). When you've reached the end, hold for three seconds (7). Do two sets of each.

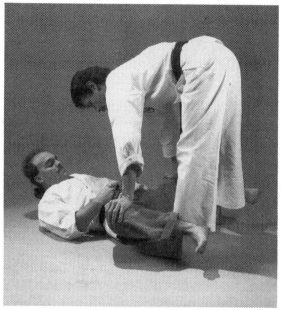

1

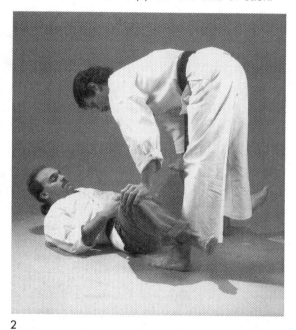

2

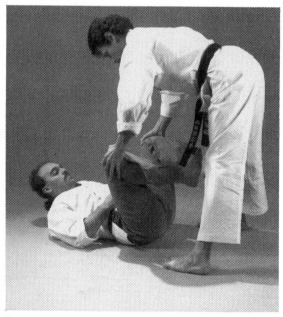

5

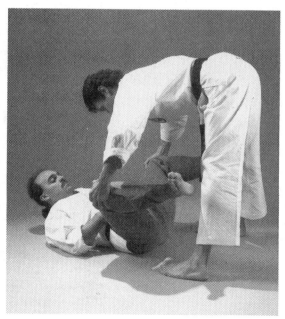

6

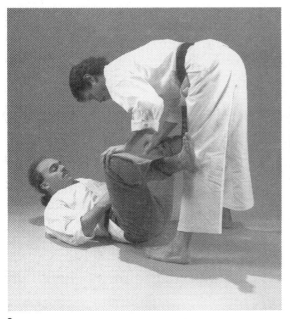

3

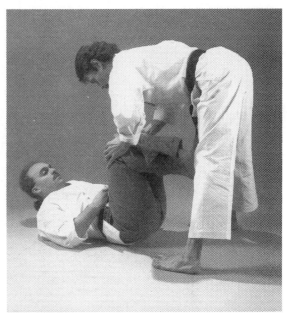

4

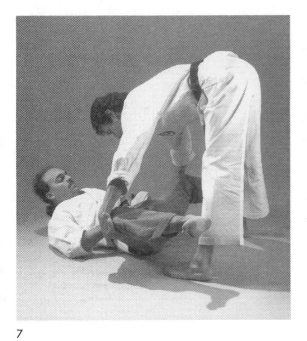

7

Get on your back, with your legs up and your feet together (1). Start to open your legs as your partner resists (2). Keep opening (3). Go as far as you can and hold for three seconds (4). From that position, start to close your legs (5). Again your partner resists. Keep trying to close your legs (6). When you reach the end, hold for three seconds (7). Do two sets of each.

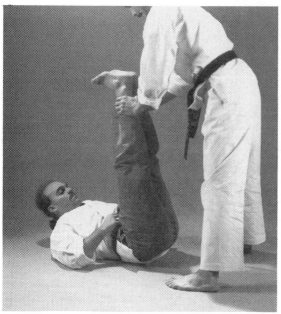

1

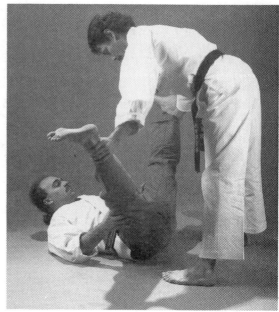

2

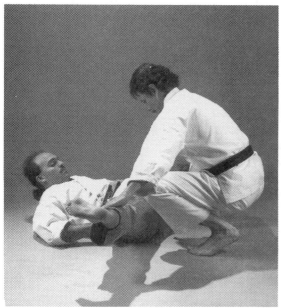

5

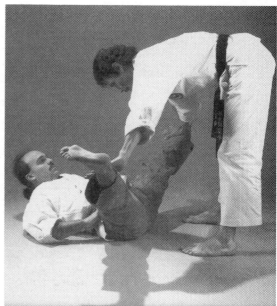

6

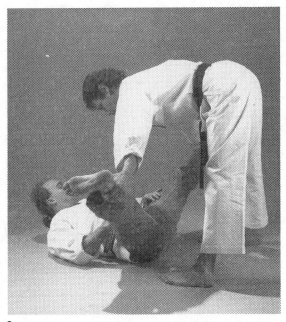

3

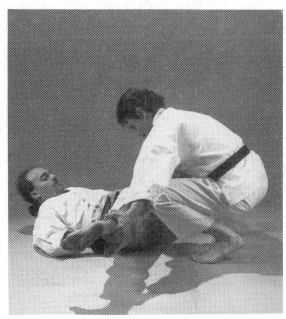

4

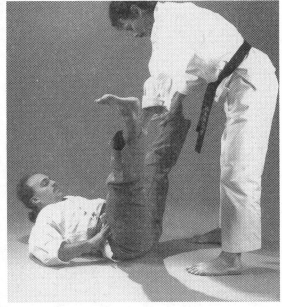

7

Get on your back and hold up your left leg (1). Your partner will be holding the leg. Try to pull the leg down as your partner resists (2). Keep going down (3). When you reach the end, hold for three seconds (4).

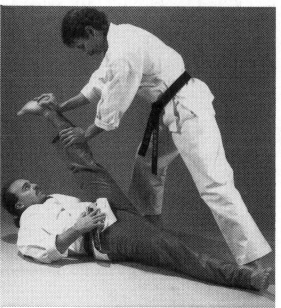

1

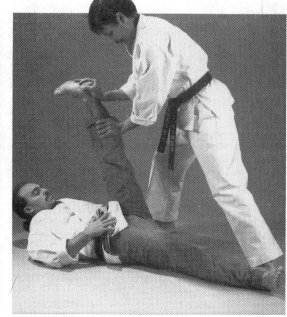

2

Lie on the ground and throw your leg up in a side kick position (1). Try to pull your leg down (2). Keep trying, fighting your partner's resistance (3). When you've reached the end hold for three seconds (4).

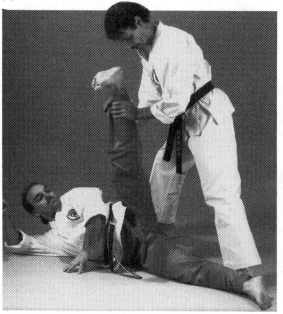

1

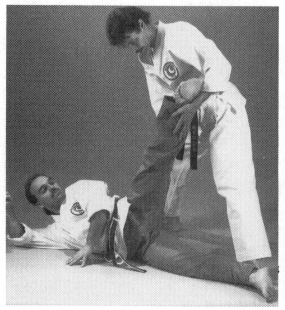

2

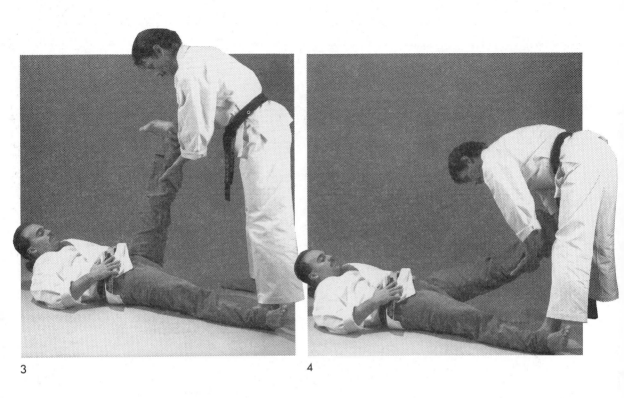

3

4

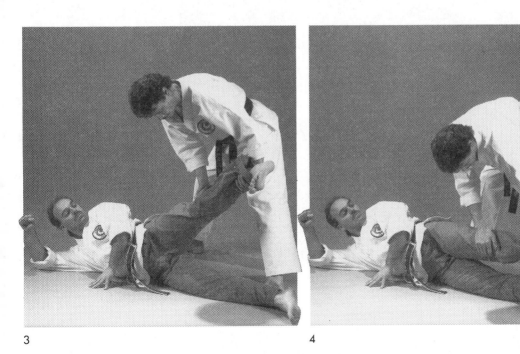

3

4

Standing, your left leg is in front, three feet from your right (1). Lean down and touch your head to your shin (2). Hold for ten seconds. Stand and twist to your right leg (3). Lean down and touch your head to your shin (4). Twist to your left and lean over (5). Touch your head to your shin. Twist to the right and do the same thing (6). Twist to your left, do a full split and touch your head to your shin (7). Twist to the right and do the same thing (8).

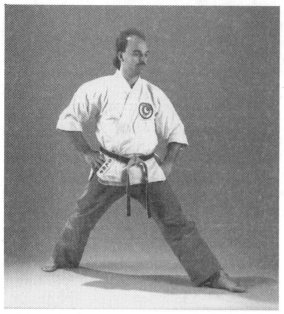

1

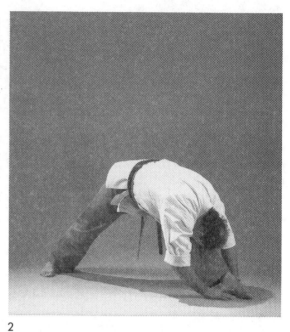

2

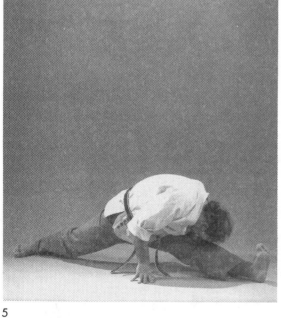

5

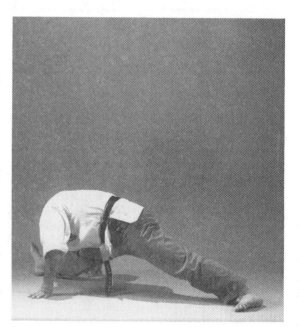

6

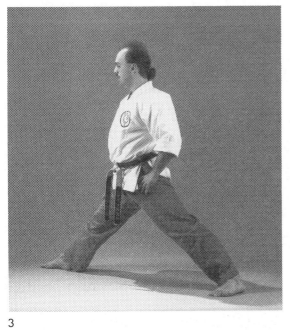

3

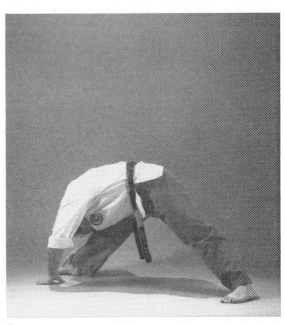

4

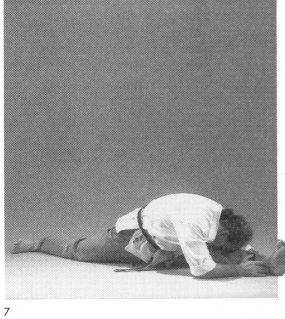

7

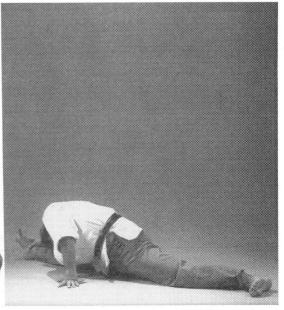

8

You are in a half-splits position, with your hands on the ground (1). Move your hips forward and hold for five seconds (2). Move your hips backward and hold for five seconds (3).

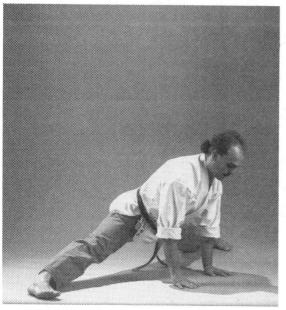

1

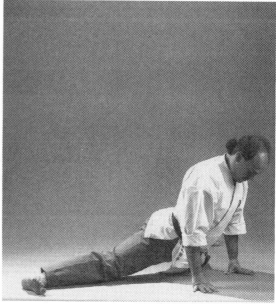

2

Partner Stretch

While assuming a frog position, your hips are straight and your knee and left leg are in a side kick posture (1). Your partner pushes on your hips (2). Go as far back as you can and hold for five seconds. Do three repetitions.

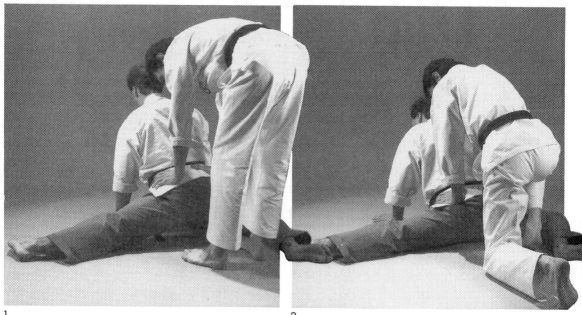

1

2

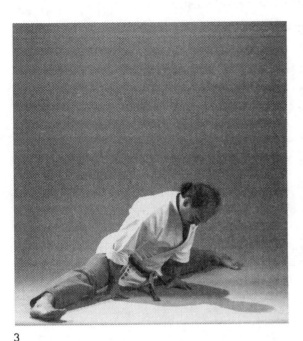

3

This exercise stretches the left knee in the front kick position (1). The partner behind keeps your back in position, while the partner in front lifts your knee. Always do both sides and hold for ten seconds.

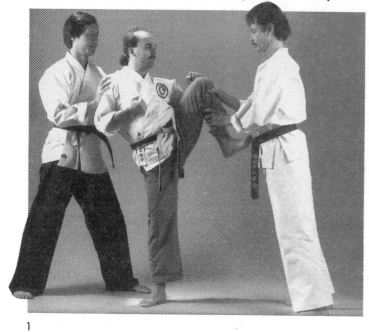

1

Stretch the left knee into a side kick position (1). The partner behind keeps your back in position, while the partner in front lifts your knee (2). Always do both sides and hold for ten seconds.

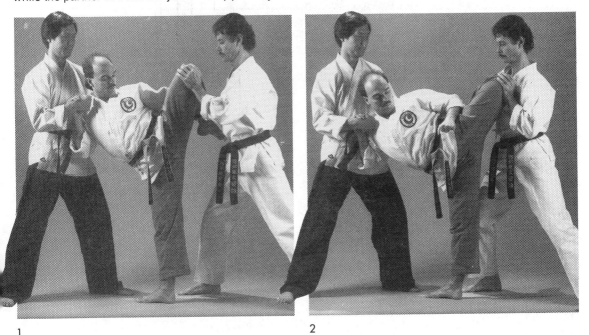

1

2

STRETCHING'S ADVANCED STAGE

This is the stage in your stretching regimen that separates those who merely perform the routines and those who use the techniques to reach their maximum potential.

The advanced stage is limited to athletes who can either do the splits or are very close to succeeding. If you are to take full advantage of these sequences, you must always push as hard as you can and go as far as you can. Now I don't mean you should risk injury at the expense of reaching a new level, but at the same time there should be a concerted effort to get everything you can from the stretching exercise.

This stage is also where the bulk of one- and two-partner stretching is introduced. There are so many levels of stretching excellence available to those who utilize partners in their routine. The difference between working by yourself and working with one or more partners is measured in degrees of accomplishment. A partner can help you go that extra step by pushing or applying pressure to a specific body part. He can push forward or backward, side to side. Just that little extra can take you to new stretching heights. As much as we hate to admit it, we don't always push ourselves to the limit. As such, we risk not reaching our maximum potential. But with one or more partners applying pressure, pushing you past what you considered unreachable limits, you'll find that the advanced stretching stage is a new and exciting world.

Despite the challenge of these exercises, there's very little risk of injury — if everyone is correctly doing his job. When I'm stretching, I'm not looking at my partner. I'm concentrating on a specific muscle. Conversely, my partner will watch my face and listen to my breathing pattern. If I begin to show pain or my breathing becomes irregular, then it is time to release pressure. Another easy way to show you've had enough is to tap the floor or your partner's shoulder several times.

Sit on the floor and assume a butterfly position (1). Your partner is standing. Try to slowly lift him with your legs (2). Two repetitions equal one set.

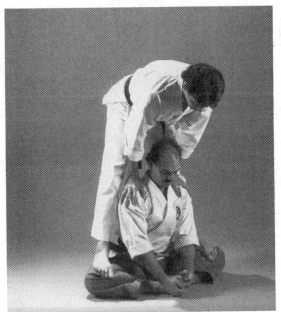

1

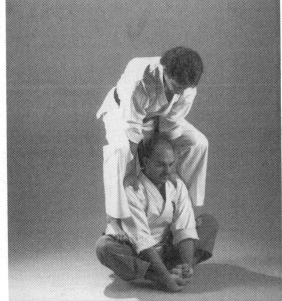

2

Lie on your back with your feet together. Your partner is holding your hands (1). Your partner steps on your left thigh (2). Then he steps on your right thigh (3). You lift as high as you can (4). Then you slowly let him down (5). Two reps equal one set.

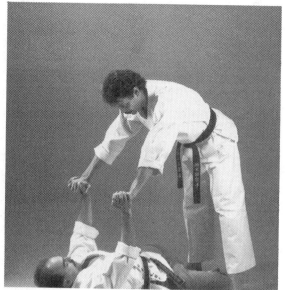

1

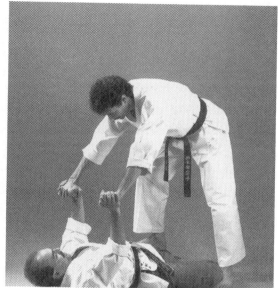

2

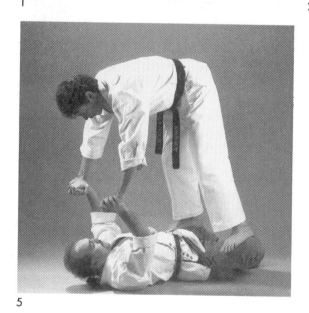

5

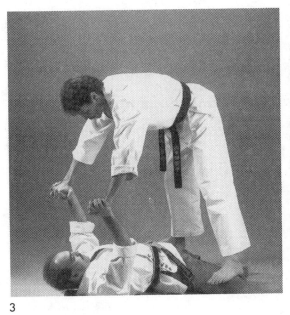

3

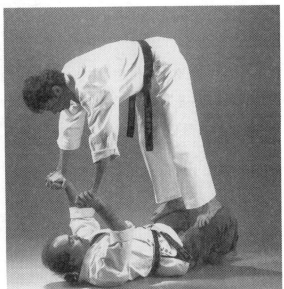

4

Lie on your back with your knees up and in a straight line with the hips (1). Your partner steps on your left thigh (2). Then he steps on your right thigh (3). You lift him as high as you can (4) and then slowly let him down (5). Do two reps.

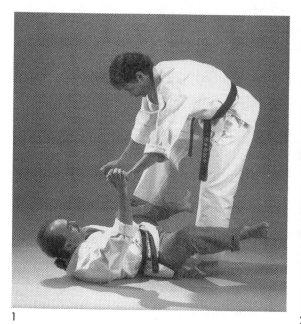

1

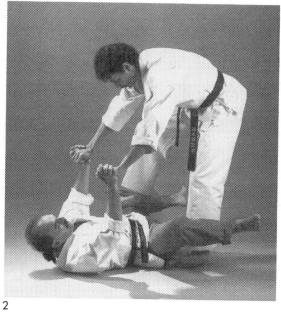

2

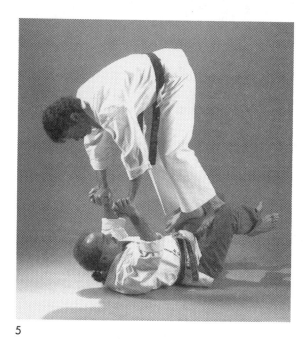

5

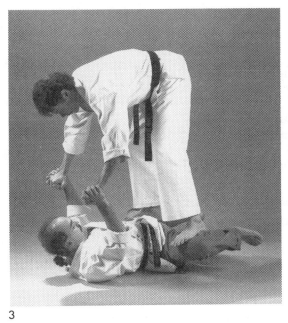

3

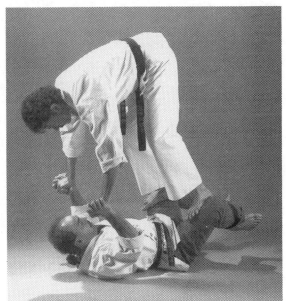

4

Assume a frog position, with your knees and hips straight. Your partner stands on your hips (1). Hold only once for three seconds.

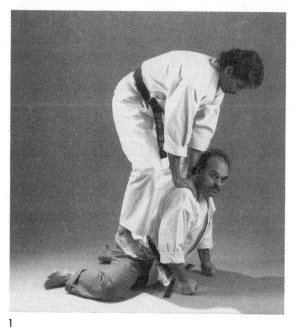

1

Standing, extend your leg in a left front kick position (1). Your partner holds your leg. Bend your supporting leg so the knee is at a 45-degree angle (2). Extend your supporting leg as your partner steps back (3). Stretch as far as you can.

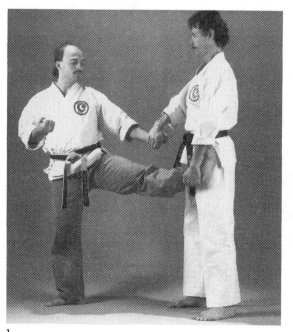

1

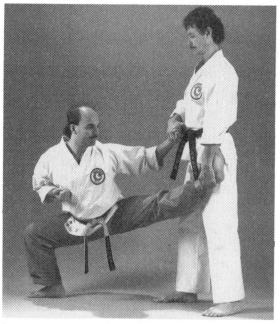

2

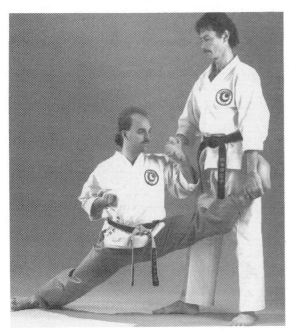

3

Standing, extend your leg in a left side kick position (1). Your partner holds your leg. Bend the supporting leg so the knee is at a 45-degree angle (2). Extend your supporting leg as your partner steps back (3). Stretch as far as you can.

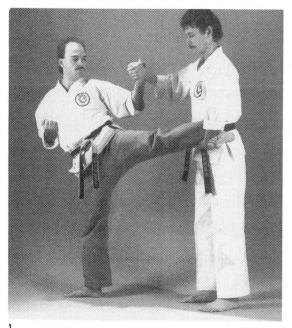

1

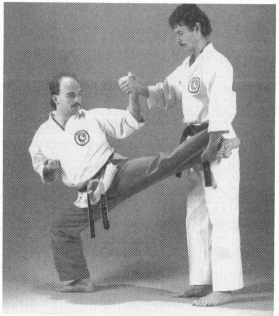

2

Standing, extend your right leg in a back kick position (1). Your partner holds your leg. Bend your supporting leg so the knee is at a 45-degree angle (2). Extend your supporting leg as your partner steps back (3). Step as far as you can.

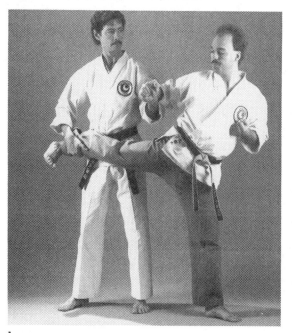

1

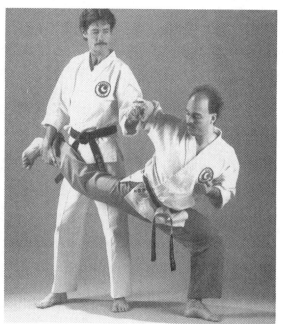

2

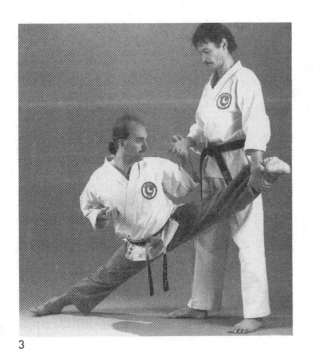

3

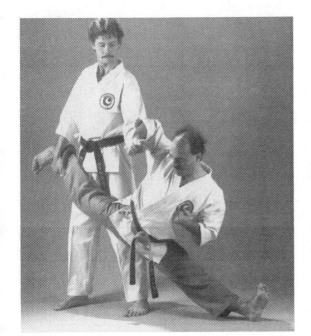

3

Extend your leg in a left front kick position (1). Your partner grabs your leg and holds the left hand. As your partner begins to move away, try to keep your balance (2). Slowly allow yourself to reach the floor. Don't just drop the leg (3). Your partner keeps your upper body straight (4). Now twist your body to the left (5). Pull your body backward (6). Now push down your hips (7).

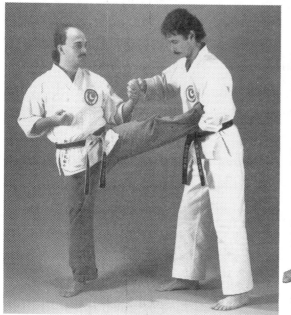

1

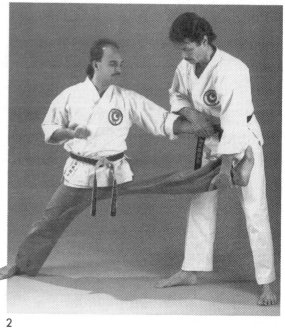

2

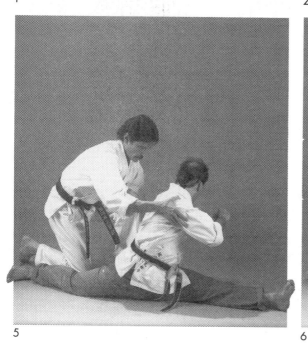

5

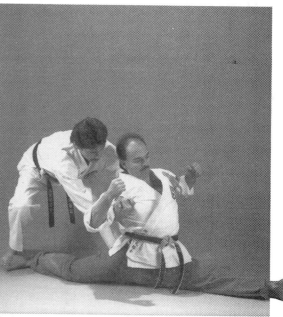

6

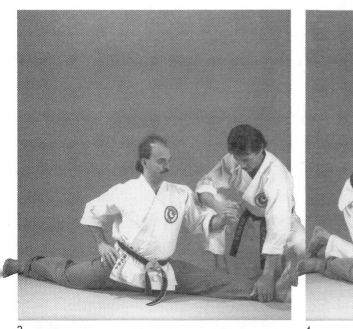

3

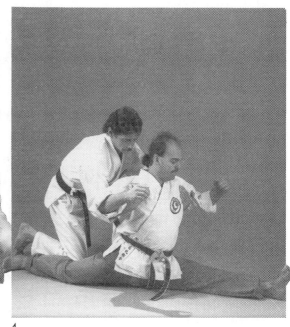

4

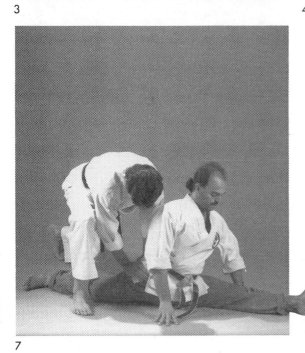

7

Extend your left leg in a left side kick position (1). Your partner grabs your left and holds the left hand. As your partner begins to move away, try to keep your balance (2). Slowly allow yourself to reach the floor. Don't just drop the leg (3). Now your partner pulls you up a little bit (4). Then he places both knees on your buttocks (5). Your partner pushes forward as far as he can (6). Hold for five seconds. Drop down as far as you can (7). Hold for five seconds (8).

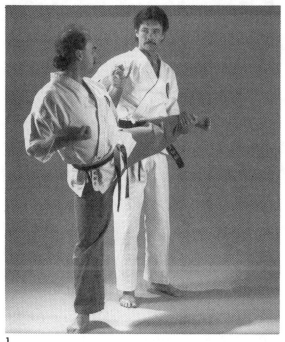

1

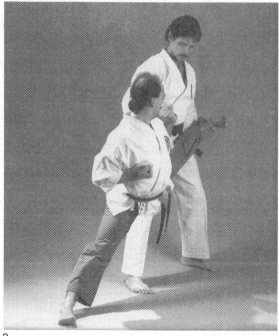

2

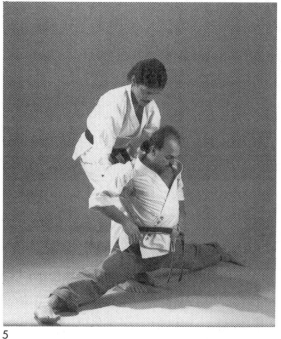

5

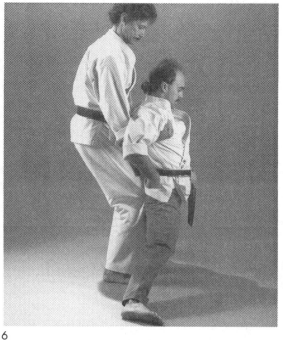

6

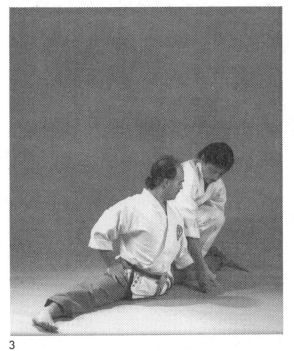

3

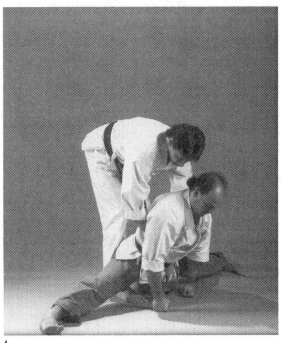

4

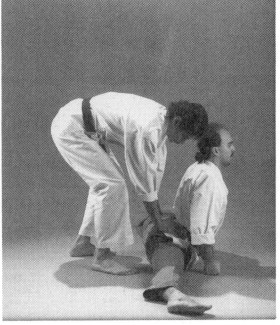

7

8

Assume a front stance, with your partner's right leg on your shoulder (1). Start moving into a back stance as your partner stretches (2). Go as far as you can while maintaining balance (3).

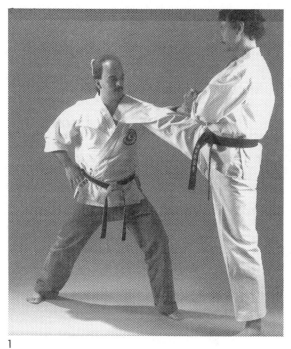

1

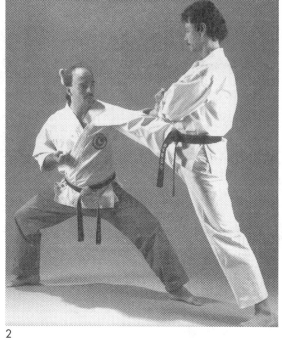

2

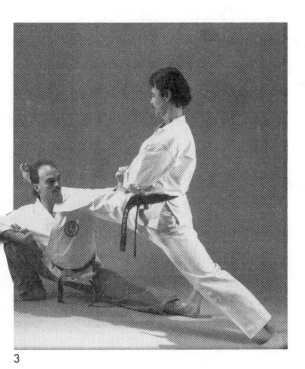

3

Your right knee is on the floor and your left leg is in a side kick position (1). As your partner begins to lift, he simultaneously holds down your body (2). Open your hips to the maximum level (3). Now return and relax (4). Now open your hips again to the maximum level (5).

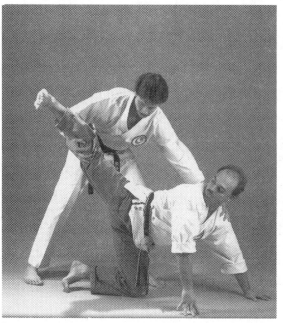

1

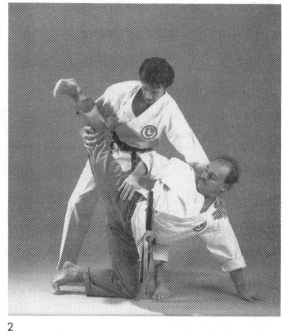

2

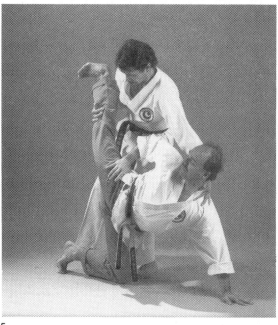

5

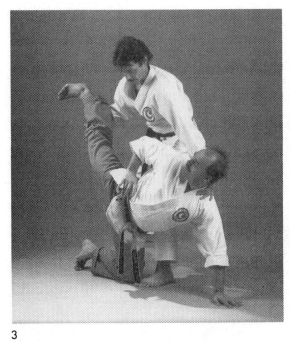

3

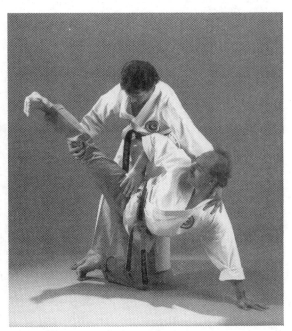

4

Splits Beyond

Stand with one foot on a phone book (1). Drop into a full split (2). Go as far as you can and hold for ten seconds (3-4). Attempt the same exercise with two phone books (5). And then three phone books (6).

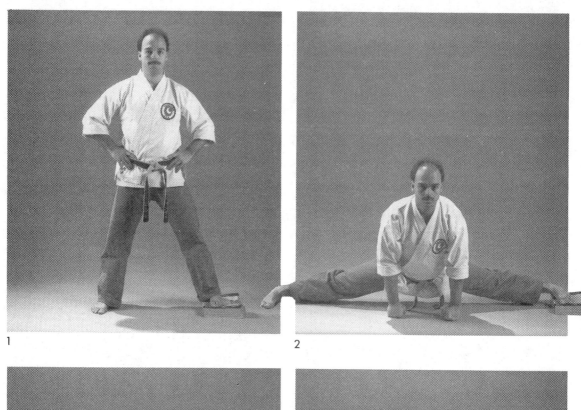

1

2

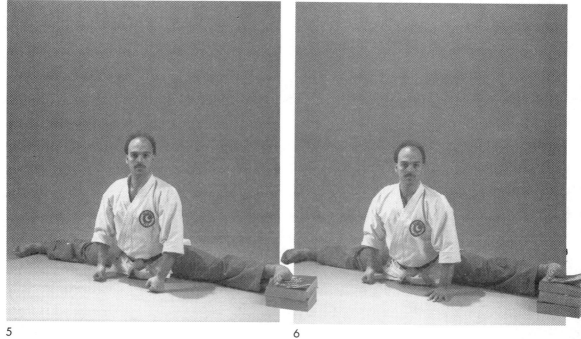

5

6

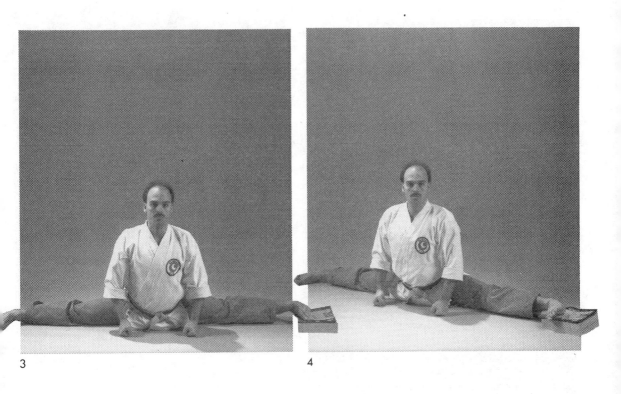

3

4

Legs Conditioning

Assume a front stance (1). Begin lifting your leg straight (2). Keep going up (3). Go as far as you can (4). Return to the original position (5).

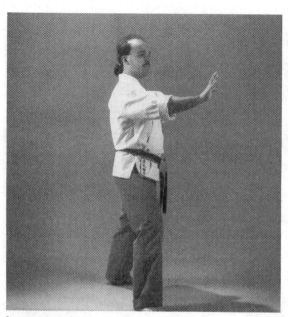

1

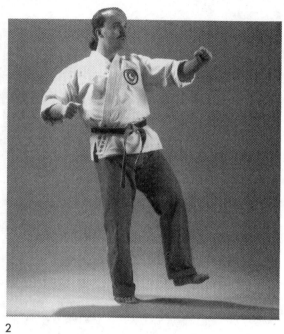

2

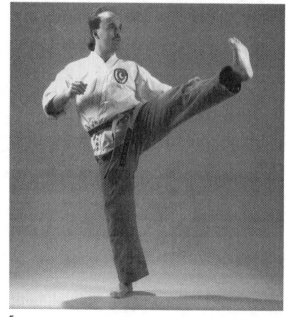

5

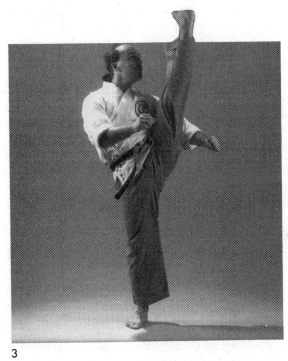

3

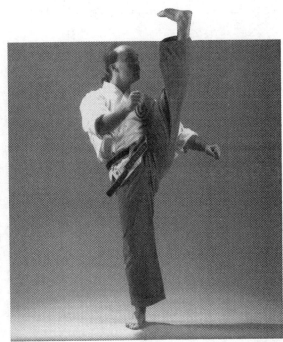

4

Assume a right front stance position (1). Start twisting your hips and turning to the right (2). Lift your left leg to the right side (3). Keep going up on the right side (4). Begin moving to the left with your leg at the same level (5). Move your leg down (6). Return to the original position and you've come full circle (7).

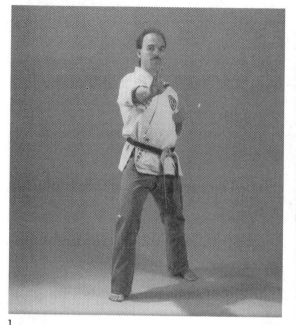

1

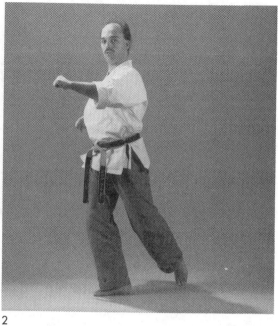

2

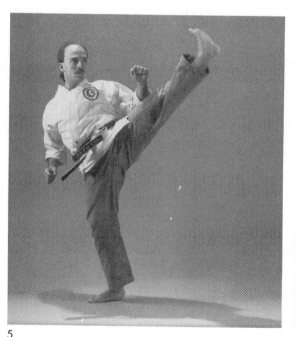

5

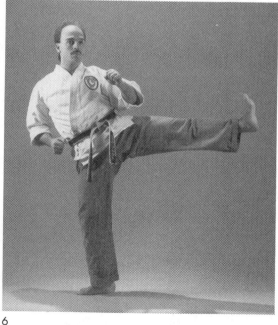

6

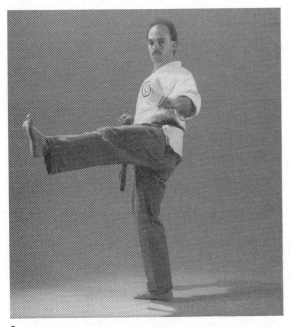

3

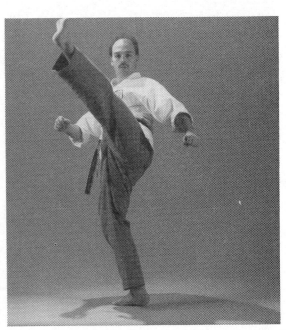

4

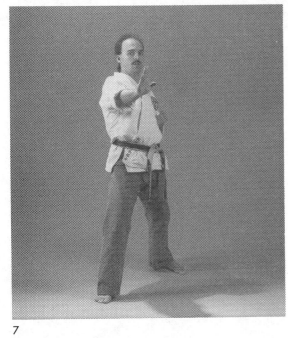

7

You right leg is back and your left leg extended (1). Twist into a deep right front stance (2). Now extend your right leg while your left is back (3). Twist into a deep left leg front stance (4).

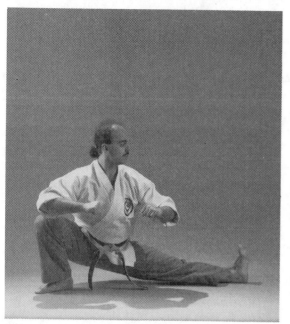
1

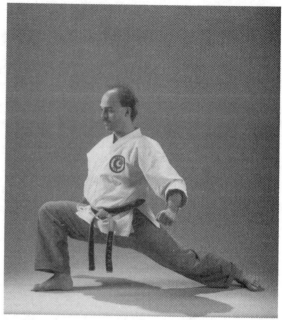
2

Assume a deep front stance position (1). Move all the way back (2-3).

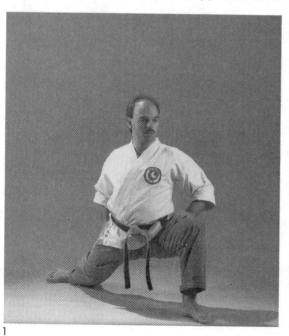
1

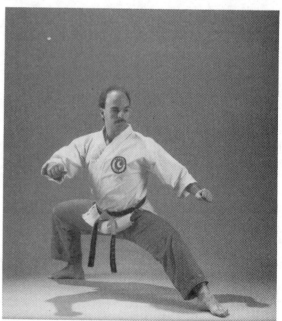
2

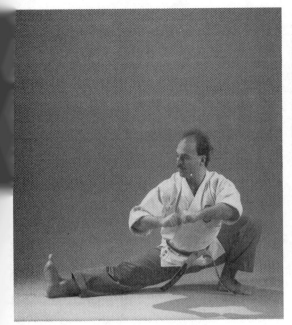

3

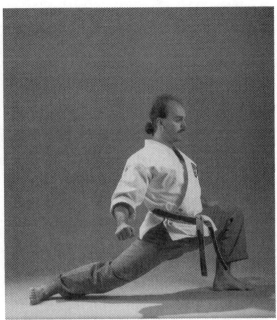

4

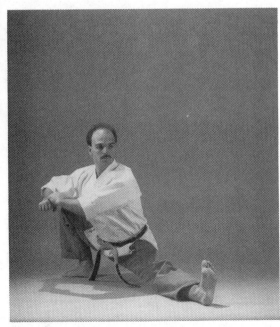

3

Face your partner in a front stance. You are holding his left hand (1). Start lifting the right leg (2). Be sure to maintain your balance (3). Go as far as you can and then return to your original position (4).

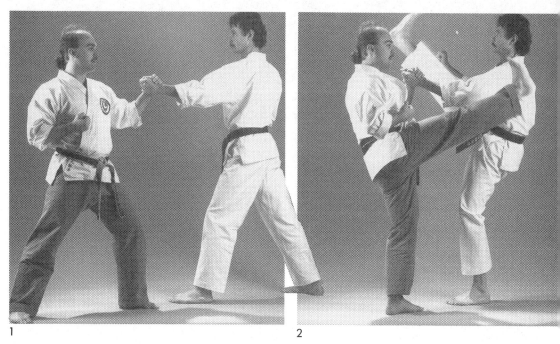

1

2

Face your partner, with your hand in his (1). Lift your left leg into a side kick position (2). Go as far as you can (3).

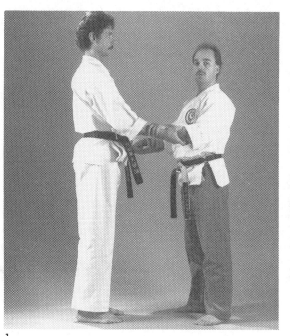

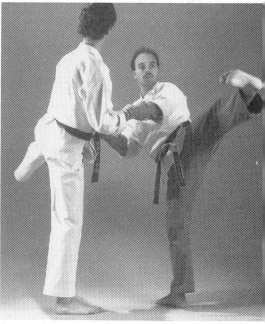

1

2

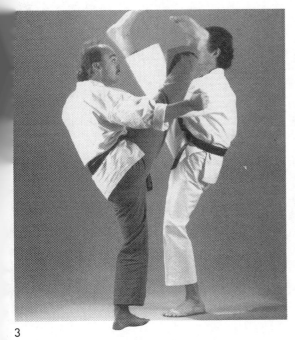

3

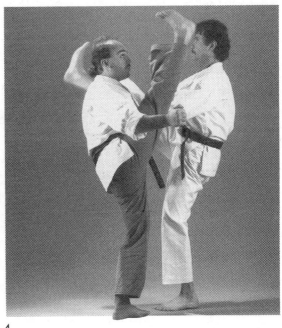

4

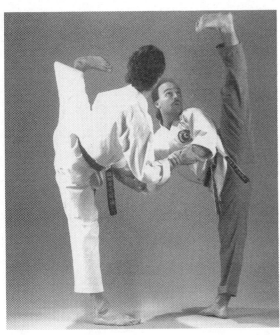

3

Face your partner, with your hand in his (1). Lift your right leg back (2). Keep going (3). Go as far as you can then return to the original position (4).

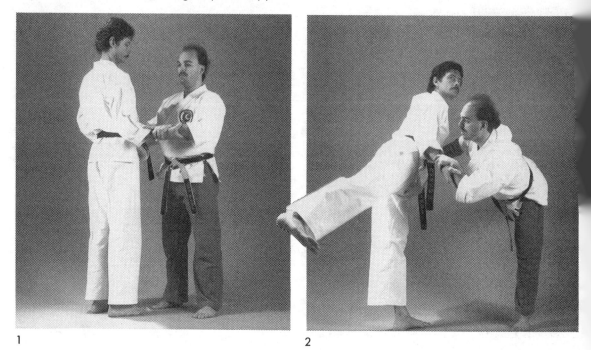

1   2

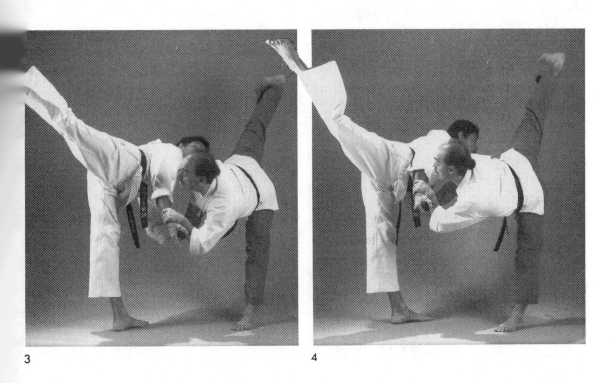

3

4

Stand with feet a shoulder-width apart (1). Go down (2). Your arms should be at chest level (3). Start going up (4). Lift left knee (5). Perform a front kick (6). Keep the knee up (7). Return to first position (8). Do 20 repetitions with each leg.

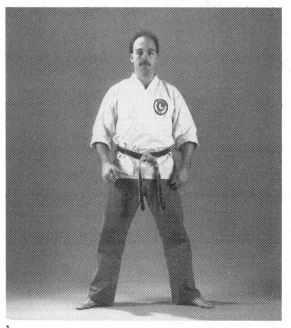

1

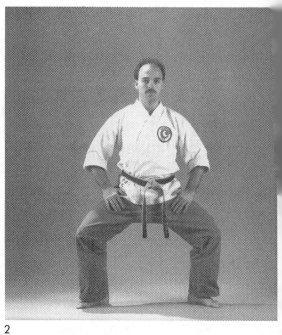

2

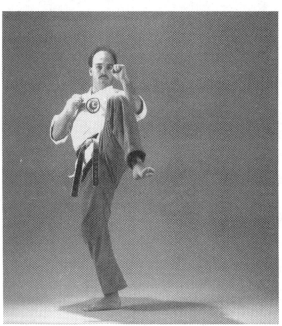

5

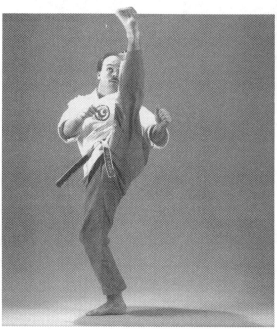

6

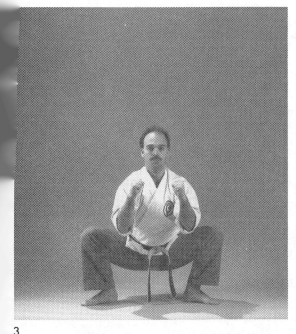

3

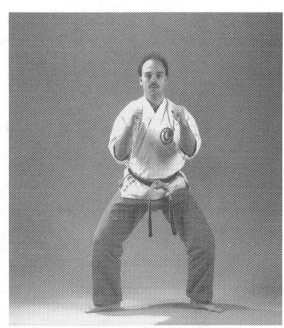

4

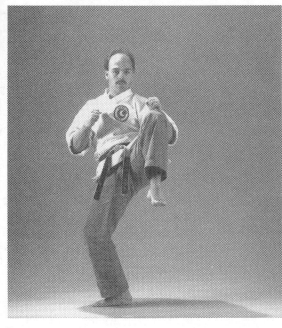

7

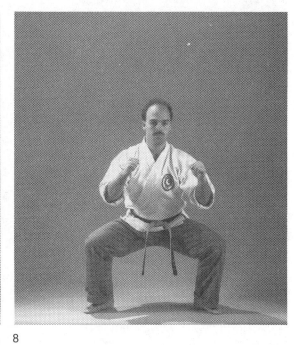

8

ABOUT
THE AUTHOR

Jean Frenette has been among the world's best-known martial artists since he won his first junior championship in Montreal, Quebec, in the mid-1970s. He followed his domination of the junior circuit by capturing the Quebec adult forms championship in 1980. He has reigned as the overall Canadian forms champion since 1981.

A Montreal native, Jean has been rated in the top ten in forms competition in the United States since 1983, twice garnering the coveted top position. Voted to the *Inside Karate* Hall of Fame in 1988, Jean has won hundreds of tournament forms grand championships. His proudest achievements include a world forms title at the 1987 World Amateur Karatedo Organization (WAKO) World Championships in Munich, West Germany, the 1985 Bermuda Invitational Open Forms Grandchampionships, and the 1986 South African Open Forms Grandchampionship.

Jean's amazing talents have led to numerous roles on screen and in television. Among his 31 screen credits are work on all six *Police Academy* movies, *Sadie and Son* with Debbie Reynolds, and stuntwork on *Speed Zone* (formerly *Cannonball Run III*). He also has appeared as a guest on several Canadian soap operas and "Knighthawk," an action series on the Fox Television network.

Currently president of WAKO Canada, Jean is considered one of the world's top seminar performers. In addition to being booked several years in advance, Frenette in the coming year will hold seminars in Russia, Europe, Asia, and Australia, as well as the United States and Canada.

A member of the prestigious Transworld Oil Karate Team, Jean recently completed a three-part stretching series for Panther Productions. Despite just being introduced to the martial arts marketplace, the tapes already are among Panther's bestsellers.

Jean would like to thank these instructors and coaches for helping him in his martial arts career: Maxime Mazaltarim, Yoshinao Nanbu, Chuck Merriman and Shigeru Kimura.

Jean presently runs a martial arts school in Montreal, Quebec, Canada. Anyone wishing to write Jean Frenette can contact him at 1189 du Perche, Boucherville, Quebec, Canada J4B 6V3.